THE PERSISTENT SPIRAL

The Ancient History of Lyme Disease and Tick-borne Co-Infections

M.M. DRYMON PhD

The Persistent Spiral. © Copyright 2018
by M.M. Drymon
All rights reserved.

Library of Congress Cataloging Data
Drymon, M.M.
The Persistent Spiral:
The Ancient History of Lyme Disease and Tick-borne Infections
p. cm.
Includes bibliographical references
ISBN 978-1717909008
1.Lyme Disease 2. Tick Borne Disease 3. Infectious Disease
4. Medical History 5. World History

Second Edition

Library of Congress Control Number:
2017917521

www.facebook.com/lymehistory
Published by The Landscape History Institute
South Portland, Maine 04106
United State of America

CONTENTS

INTRODUCTION
7
ONE BITE- PATHOGENS
17
THE PERSISTENT SPIRAL
33
ANCIENT IMMUNITY
53
EXPERIENCING SYMPTOMS
73
QUESTING FOR DINOSAURS
79
NANDY-THE NEANDERTHAL WITHIN
87
LANDSCAPES ON FIRE
99
THE CRADLE OF LYME DISEASE- BORRELIA IN THE BONE
111
CHILDREN OF THE GRASS
121
THE YELLOW EMPEROR- BORRELIA IN CHINA
137
ÖTZI- BORRELIA ON ICE
149
CHICKEN- BORRELIA FOR THE BIRDS!
153
ROMANS, CATS AND BARTONELLA
157
QUESTING FOR CRUSADERS- BORRELIA IN THE MOUTH
165
WHEN ENGLAND SWEAT- BABESIA
171
CONCLUSIONS
193
REFERENCES
201

FIGURES
1. Worldwide Distribution of Lyme Disease.
2. Size of *Ixodes* ticks.
3. How ticks absorb moisture.
4. Before and After a Blood Meal.
5. Schematic of Ecology of Lyme Disease.
6. Last Glacial Maxima and Present Vegetation.
7. Structure of a Borrelia spirochete.
8. Maximum Clade Credibility Tree.
9. Spirochetes, blebs and persisters.
10. Bull's Eye Rash.
11. Bell's Palsy.
12. Age and Sex distribution.
13. Seasonal Pattern of Lyme Disease in New England.
14. Summary of landscape of Lyme disease risk.
15. Modern Protection recommendations.
16. A Denisovan Bone Fragment.
17. A Chromosome Pair.
18. Cells involved in the Immune System.
19. How HIV infects a cell
20. The Tick/Mammal interface.
21. Anaplasma.
22. Ancient *Paleoborrelia.*
23. Fossilized Blood with *Babesia.*
24. 100 million year old Rickettsia, Rocky Mountain Spotted Fever.
25. A 'Neanderthal child.'
26. World Map of Y-DNA Haplogroups
27. A Bonfire.
28. Tick Habitat Drag Results.
29. Long-term burning as tick control.
30. North America during Glaciation.
31. Knee osteoarthritis.
32. The Four Horsemen of the Apocalypse.
33. The Great Yamnaya Migration.
34. Scythian on Horseback.
35. Kurgen Burial Mound.
36. The White Horse, Wiltshire, U.K.
37. The Yellow Emperor.
38. Distribution of Tick-borne Infections in China.
39. Ötzi .
40. Woodcut of *Gallus Indicus auritus tridactylus*
41. Cats and Witches having fun
42. *Bartonella*- Cat Scratch Rash.
43. Crusader Siege.
44. Crusader Routes through Europe.
45. Anne Boleyn by Hans Holbein the younger.
46. Queen Elizabeth hunting.
47. Catherine of Aragon as a teenager.
48. Catherine of Aragon as a middle aged women.

TABLES
1. Chart of Afflicted Over Time.
2. Lyme Disease Characteristics.
3. Neanderthal Disease Packages.

Dedicated to those,
past and present,
who have suffered
from Lyme Disease and
Tick-borne Co-Infections.

INTRODUCTION

"It's likely that many ailments in human history for which doctors had no explanation have been caused by tick-borne disease."
                                             Dr. George Poinar, Jr.

This work is the result of a long journey that I began in 1994 with a short walk in the woods. I was bitten by an *Ixodes* tick that was carrying the spiral shaped bacteria called *Borrelia burgdorferi* in its gut. The tick hopped on, attached behind my knee, took a blood meal, and the spirochetes entered my bloodstream. I soon began to suffer from the spectrum of symptoms that is known as Lyme disease.

It was a life altering experience. Chained to my bed by severe fatigue, as a consummate historian, I began to wonder if people had been similarly afflicted like this in the past. How did they cope in pre-antibiotic times? It is hard enough in this Era of "Modern Medicine." If you acquire Lyme disease and remain sick after the prescribed length of antibiotic treatment- you are a modern medical pariah. How would it have been in the past. Were people told that it was "all in their head?" Would they be looked upon as afflicted or considered malingerers by their social group's belief systems?

Recognizing that past belief systems, even those based upon magic, were considered real by the people experiencing their lived lives requires a move away from the Cartesian dichotomies of modern logic. I knew that interactions with deadly as well as nuisance illnesses and food deprivations in the past had created cultural memories that are still interwoven into the fabric of our modern social systems as well and astoundingly, can even be found within our personal biology. The field of epigenetics, which studies how forces outside of our actual DNA genome have changed the very structure of our genetic makeup, is a relatively new but expanding discipline. It sits at an intersection between biology and history.

The famines suffered during the childhood of a grandfather have been found to affect the genes of not only his children but his grandchildren as well. Another study has found that exposure to and survival from a pox infection during the 14th Century A.D. made the descendants of its European survivors immune to the ravages of HIV infections in the twentieth-century. Another recent study has found that epigenetic information can influence some species genetic make-up for up to fourteen generations. It may last a lot longer-humans have been found to carry inherited Neanderthal immune reactions that may have been acquired hundreds of thousands of years ago.

I wondered how far back Lyme disease's influence would go. I developed the hypothesis that : It is an OLD affliction that has helped shape human cultures since pre-historic times. I would look for Lyme related genetic evidence, cultural practices, and descriptions of symptoms that had occurred in the past remembering that past cultures responded to and defined their human experiences in ways that made sense within their own particular times and places. I would apply modern research as well as my personal experience of the affliction of Lyme disease to the past.

This study uses the concept of pathocenosis that was first conceptualized by Mirko Grmek, a prominent medical historian of the early twentieth century. Grmek used a temporal and spatial approach to understanding the dynamics of the spread of disease infections and pathogen interdependency. He believed that changing environmental, social, and technological factors played a role in disease emergence, establishment, and sometimes disappearance- over time in any particularly defined population within any defined space. This creates a variety of epidemiological patterns in different places. I have added in genetics as an important but changing factor into his theory.

Grmek believed that the dynamics of infectious disease were also strongly influenced by the relationships between a community of interacting infectious agents that are present at any point in time within any human body within any social group living within any particular space. Grmek examined the historical progression of

diseases across Europe over time, beginning with the replacement of leprosy by plague and ending with Acquired Immune Deficiency Syndrome.

I see Lyme disease as a constellation of human pathogens, centered upon the *Borrelia* spirochete but including many co-infections and other factors. Ticks are second only to mosquitoes as vectors of pathogens throughout history but this role has been vastly under-recognized. The microbial pathogens they transmit may include protozoa, helminths, fungi, bacteria, and viruses-a literal infective soup. Transferred helminths[worm like parasites] can harbor many other pathogens-giving them an extra layer of cellular protection against the human immune system.

My thinking has also been influenced by the work of the French bacteriologist, Charles Nicolle, who proposed a dynamic concept of the "birth, life, and death of infectious diseases" to highlight the continuity and dynamics of the pathogenic domain of any given host population at any given time. Nicolle is important because he was the first researcher to propose the concept of "asymptomatic infection" which is crucial to understanding interactive causalities and the sudden appearance of certain diseases under particular circumstances, which can be applied to Lyme disease.

Since the publication of my book *Disguised as the Devil* in 2008, in which I linked the symptoms of witch affliction and characteristics of the western witch with Lyme disease,there has been change. In 2008, Lyme disease was still considered a NEW disease that had been discovered by the best minds that modern medicine could produce. Since then the antiquity of Lyme disease has come to be an accepted concept. However, the idea that Lyme disease is a difficult, life altering affliction has yet to be accepted. You still don't "get it until you get it!" The concept that people suffered from Lyme disease in the past has yet to be accepted. The idea that people living in Salem, Massachusetts in 1692 may have displayed identifying symptoms is still considered "farfetched," to quote one critic.

Identifying Katherine of Aragon as suffering from Lyme disease and *Babesia* will probably elicit a similar disdain. The infection of Ötzi, the ice mummy, has been somewhat accepted, although some Lyme Activists wonder how Lyme can be found in a 5000 year old body when the diagnostic tests are so poor that it is almost impossible to test positive for living human beings. The fact that *Borrelial* DNA was found within his body is hard to dispute, although some have tried. Some have a simple and narrow definition for Lyme disease. In the simple and narrow definition, Lyme disease is a geographically limited tick-borne infection, is hard to catch, is easy to treat, and goes away after a few handfuls of antibiotics are consumed. Those who disagree, especially female Lyme Activists, as disdained as anti-science and anti-vaxers. My experience, along with that of many people within the [2013 annual] thirty six percent treatment failure rate, does not fit this model.

In this work, I use a complex and broad definition for Lyme disease. I use the broader definition described by the 'Lyme Denialists' as a belief that Lyme disease is "insidious, ubiquitous, difficult to diagnose, and almost incurable,"(Auwaerter,et al., 2011) a long lasting and complex infection with inflammation and autoimmune reactions that can affect multiple organ systems. It has also been around for a long time, and the afflicted may exhibit symptoms that vary, depending on where in the world your inherited immune system was being trained in the past

As a lived experience, many subscribe to the broad definition. Even Dr. Todd Murray, one of the children who participated in Dr. Allen Steere's original Connecticut Lyme study, still suffers from Lyme-related symptoms four decades later (Daley, Dec.3,2013)! It is a spectrum of: symptoms, persistent infection, tick-borne and opportunistic co-infections that causes a complex interactive infection. *Borrelia* is a pathogen that has learned to suppress and evade the human immune system in numerous ways.

This broad definition has scientific validity and is supported by an overwhelming amount of research. The symptoms of Lyme disease are dermatological, arthritic, and neuropsychiatric. If not identified and treated early, Lyme disease can develop into a chronic, life altering, and in some instances disabling or fatal

medical problem. Chronic Lyme disease is associated with extremely poor quality of life and increased risk of suicide (*Bangor Daily News*, Bill Chinnock Obituary, September 25, 2008).

Lyme disease may have been labeled and understood as a variety of differently named diseases in the past. The affliction of Lyme disease and co-infections may have included symptoms linked to witches and witchcraft, the sweating sickness, madness, lameness, soldier's heart, rheumatism, summer sickness, neurasthenia, and currently, chronic fatigue, multiple sclerosis, and fibromyalgia. Even in the past, people would have been infected not just with *Borrelia* but with an array of other tick borne pathogens.

When I went looking for Lyme disease in Pre-enlightenment Europe, I kept finding witches. Witchcraft accusations and afflictions appear in the historic records during a distinct late Medieval and Early Modern time period in almost the identical geographical areas where people are plagued with Lyme disease today. This work serves as a prequel covering the time that includes between the emergence of the *Borrelia* bacteria as an organism, the development of the tick as a blood seeking entity, and the time period leading up to the establishment of European colonies in the Americas after 1492.

Prehistoric epidemics shaped history in ways that we have yet to understand but they still influence how we cope with pathogens. We are the descendants of our ancestors, including those bits of genetic stardust we inherited from the Neanderthals. The diseases that early humans confronted during their lives shaped our genes. We have also inherited some of the epigenetic biological processes that were developed in response to diseases long ago. Human societies have been confronted by several disease driven apocalypses in the near past that are well documented and others that occurred before recorded history have been found by advances in the study of DNA.

Geneticists have recorded the sudden "disappearance" of various haplotypes in particular areas, have traced human migration around the world, have also found that most cats in western Europe had Roman roots, and that chickens may have

been brought to South America before Columbus sailed the blue. *Flaviviruses* have been traced all the way from Africa, through Eurasia, to North America. They probably left a wave of Neanderthal and human corpses in their wake along the way.

Our nursery rhymes still warn that a "pocket full of posies" will not save us from the Black Death because eventually "we all fall down" and that opening a window may bring "influenza." Smallpox was an often lethal, scar inducing opponent, accomplishing the near annihilation of some human groups. The scientific discovery of a life saving vaccination spread around the world [created originally by the ancient Chinese], while the eighteenth century fad for decorative scar concealing face patches was popular in France and England all relate to this scourge.

Less deadly diseases, however, may have even greater cultural effect than ones that kill rapidly and then depart. For a short period of time in our early modern history, enough people were afflicted by a constellation of symptoms:the appearance of pins stuck into their flesh, "devil's marks" on their skin, seizures, bell's palsy, the sudden onset of lameness and other features that were blamed on witchcraft.

These symptoms helped set off the Great Witch Hunts of Europe and led to the Salem Witch Trials in North America, where the society was in the middle of warfare. I have attributed some of the symptoms associated with witchcraft affliction to Lyme disease. When I looked in the tick risky pre-modern forests of the world, I kept finding Hunter-Gatherers, Soldiers, and, especially in England, Upper Class sportsmen and a few privileged women.

Culture, as used here, refers to the practices, languages, accumulated knowledge, beliefs, assumptions, and values that are passed between individuals or groups over the generations. A culture has a system of meanings and symbols that shape how people use and see the world and their place in it. It gives definition to personal and collective experience.

A pathogen like the *Borrelia* spirochete and all the tick-borne co-infections have a steady accumulative effect: the disease afflicts the humans, human biology and cultural practices respond, which in turn effects the disease, in a process which continues in an

ongoing symbiotic cycle throughout time. These effects can become so intertwined and interwoven and familiar that they reach a point of near invisibility. Social definitions have come and gone while evolving landscapes and natural eco-systems have provided an ever-changing stage for the performances of human life and experience of disease. Infection with this spiral shaped bacteria may have followed a path that has varied in virulence over time and, while people have been afflicted with Lyme disease for thousands of years, what it has been called and how the disease has been defined has varied. Looking for Lyme disease in the past requires careful detective work.

Disguised as the Devil was based upon the Lyme disease and witch research that was available when it was published in 2008. Since that time, information related to the history of Lyme disease has continued to accumulate. Much of it has tended to confirm my original hypothesis that Lyme disease is an old and culturally influential affliction. Fifteen million year old *Paleoborrelia* spirochetes were found preserved in amber by Dr. George Poinar. Genetic research has reconstructed the evolutionary history of Lyme disease clades in North America, tracing it back to over 60,000 years ago. A Neolithic case of Lyme disease infection has been found in a man whose body was preserved as an ice encased mummy. He walked this earth over five thousand years ago. He lived in an Alpine setting that would be at once both very familiar and very different from our modern world.

Ötzi straddled two forms of human society-he carried a quiver full of the arrows of a hunter-gatherer but had an agrarian diet: bacon-like preserved meat and the remains of one of the earliest of domesticated grains made up his last meal. Researchers, looking at a particular oxygen isotope to determine where the water Ötzi drank during his lifetime came from, suggests that he spent up to two months of each summer high up in the mountains above the timber line, which is consistent with the theory that he was a shepherd, going to the alpine region each summer to graze livestock. His mummified body contained the physical evidence of a violent death along with the earliest DNA evidence for a Lyme disease infection ever found.

Ötzi's copper axe may have been useful in the process of deforestation that was needed for Europe's agrarian revolution to succeed. This was a tick- risky activity. The descendants of Ötzi's culture and his G genetic Y-haplotype still walk the earth. His closest modern genetic relatives now live on the Italian island of Sardinia. The agriculturalists that had joined hunter-gatherers in Europe seem to have been afflicted by a prehistoric pandemic wave of unknown pestilence. Their Y-haplotypes completely disappear in some areas and were replaced. Europe was overwhelmed by waves of R1a and R1b genetic Y-haplotype types: horse riding, cattle herding, cannabis using pastoralists who swept in from the Eurasian steppes to fill empty spaces in the landscape. They are called the Yamnaya. Modern advances in DNA research found them hiding in plain sight- a great wave of migration previously ignored by the history books.

Later, when Europeans crossed the Atlantic Ocean, they filled in spaces that had been depopulated by another wide spread epidemic, and began chopping down trees in the 'New World.' Later in time, Agrarian landscapes succumbed to Industrialization. Pastures changed back into forests. And, just when the forests of New England and Europe had grown back, they began to be cut down once more by modern suburbia in a sprawling splotchy pattern. The affliction that we call Lyme disease emerged again in this landscape. The modern designation Lyme disease was coined for the first time in 1975. Just as there were disease influenced politics in the past, there is a modern politics of Lyme disease in the present. Public policies like federal highway construction, accelerated depreciation, and the mortgage availability of the post WWII G.I. Bill were used to create the landscape of sprawl that has come to be associated with the modern iteration of this disease.

This work can be considered to be a prequel to Disguised as the Devil, although some basic information is repeated. How important is the history of Lyme disease? It is estimated that roughly 300,000 people (approximately one percent of the U.S. population) are diagnosed with Lyme disease each year (CDC, 2013) and it could possible be as many as one million. In 2015, it was the sixth most common Nationally Notifiable disease (Conner,

2017). The outcome of Lyme Disease infection varies which has a lot to do with genetics. Some people are seropositive for Lyme Disease but remain asymptomatic. Some patients are diagnosed right away, receive antibiotics, and seem to be cured. Others display a spectrum of symptoms and outcomes. Some patients suffer from what some Activists have called LYMEAIDS. Their immune systems' reaction to the Outer Surface Protein A of *Borrelia* triggers an immune deficiency which allows normally benign viruses and mycoplasma to overgrow. Others have a hyper-responsive over reaction that causes inflammation, especially in the joints. Post sepsis-persister cells and biofilms may cause symptoms that come and go in a relapsing pattern when they are reactivated. A growing proportion of patients with Lyme disease develop debilitating symptoms that persist in the absence of a gold standard testing protocol, slow initial treatment, or following short-course antibiotic therapy.

This condition is referred to as Post-treatment Lyme disease (PTLD) or, in this book, as Chronic Lyme Disease. It is estimated that as many as thirty six percent of those diagnosed and treated for Lyme disease remain chronically ill after treatment (Aucott et al., 2013). In some rare cases, Lyme Disease overwhelms the organs and systems and can cause death. There is also a growing suicide rate among the infected. Co-Infections tend to intensify symptoms and make the patient harder to treat effectively. Lyme Disease and Tick-borne infections have had a great impact on the quality of human lives both in the past and in the present. The *Borrelia* bacteria is indeed a persistent spiral.

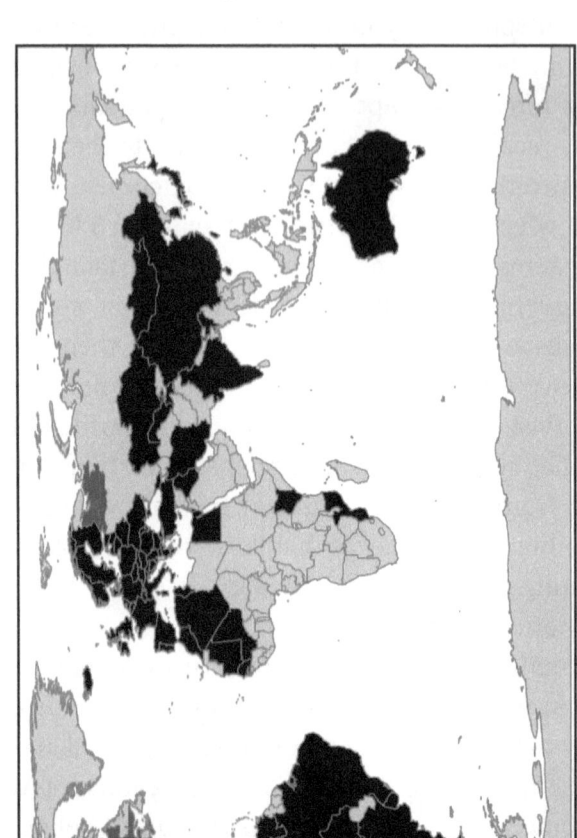

Figure 1. WORLDWIDE LYME DISEASE DISTRIBUTION. CDC.

ONE BITE- MYRIAD PATHOGENS

"...this small, vile creature may, in the future, cause the inhabitants of this land great damage"
Peter Kalm, writing about ticks while touring New England in 1749.

Lyme disease is an infection usually caused by a bacteria called *Borrelia burgdorferi*. The genus is named after the pioneering French biologist Amedee Borrel. It belongs to a spiral shaped phylum of bacteria that are called spirochetes. *Leptospirosis, Syphilis, Yaws* and *Relapsing Fever* are other diseases that are caused by spirochetes. They are distinguishable from other bacteria because of their shape and by the location of their flagella, sometimes called axial filaments, which run lengthwise along the bacteria's outer membrane creating a spiral shape. The spirochete uses the flagella to move in a twisting corkscrew spiral motion (Harmon, 2017).There are over three hundred different species and sub-species of *Borrelia*. Humans usually acquire *Borrelia* in their blood stream when they are bitten by an infected *Ixodes* tick that, while attached and drinking a blood meal, injects pathogen laden saliva into the human's bloodstream.

Ticks are arachnids, members of a class of eight legged invertebrates that also includes spiders and mites. There are two types of ticks:hard bodied and soft bodied. Diseases that commonly infect together are called co-infections and they seem

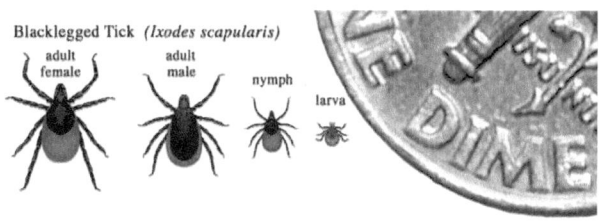

Figure 2. Size of *Ixodes* ticks. CDC

to occur as a standard, rather than exceptional, event in tick-borne infection. *Borrelia* are often accompanied within a tick's gut and/or salivary glands by a number of other bacteria, viruses, helminths, protozoa, and fungi. *Ixodes* ticks are known to carry more than two hundred and thirty seven types of bacteria and at least twenty six viruses. The most studied tick-borne co-infecting organisms accompanying Lyme disease are *Babesia, Ehrlichia/Anaplasma,* and *Powassan virus.* Additionally, the evidence supporting *Bartonella* as a tick-borne co-infection is growing (Eskow, et al. 2001). *Mycoplasm, Chlamydia Pneumoniae, Human Herpes Virus 6,* and *Epstein Barr Virus* have all also been associated with ticks (www.lyme.org).

There are many species of *Borrelia* and each is adapted to a specific tick vector; in return, each tick species has a preferred set of hosts which serve as natural reservoirs for the spirochetes. Humans are incidental hosts. Once inside a human bloodstream, *Borrelia* and/or pathogenic co-infections may compromise the immune system, which allows asymptomatic but co-existing infections like *Epstein Barr Virus* or *Mycoplasma* to become symptomatic. The combination of these various infective pathogens alters the manifestations of Lyme Disease, making it even more difficult to eradicate. A recently published survey of over three thousand patients with Chronic Lyme disease found that over fifty percent had co-infections, with thirty percent reporting more than two co-infections (Johnson, et al, 2014, Stricker and Fesler, 2017).

Due to advances in research, the tick-borne pathogens *Ehrlichia* and *Anaplasma* have been placed together into a single genus, *Anaplasma. Anaplasma phagocytophilum* causes human granulocytic anaplasmosis [HGA]. These parasitic microbes invade and occupy specific compartments within host cells, called vacuoles, that are responsible for nutrient uptake and the release of cellular waste. They infect the cells of peripheral blood- red blood cells, leukocytes and platelets. *Anaplasma* invades neutrophil cells and builds bacterial microcolonies known as morulae. *Anaplasma*

causes an increase in the secretion of IL-8, a chemoattractant that increases the phagocytosis of neutrophils.

Anaplasma was first 'discovered' in 1990, although the pathogen was known to cause veterinary disease since as early as 1932. Symptoms are flu-like and can include fever, chills, fatigue and joint pain. Anaplasmosis is a global infection, occurring in North America, most of Europe and eastern Asia. *Ixodes* ticks from are the vectors:*scapularis* in the northeastern and upper Midwestern regions of the United States; *pacificus* in the Pacific Northwest; *ricinus* in Europe and *persulcatus* in Asia (CDC, 2010).

A vector is an organism that transmits an infective pathogen from one host to another. For Lyme disease *Borrelia burgdorferi* the vector is the *Ixodes* tick. Lyme disease is today recognized by the CDC as "the leading cause of vector-borne infectious illness in the United States." The most recent CDC estimate was for a total number of 329,000 new cases per year in 2015.

Called the black legged deer tick, *Ixodes scapularis* spreads Lyme disease in the Northeastern, Mid-Atlantic, and North-Central United States. The western black legged tick, *Ixodes pacificus,* spreads the disease along the Pacific Coast of North America. In Europe, the main vector tick is *Ixodes ricinus,* and in Asia it is *Ixodes persulcatus.*

Other tick species have been found to also sometimes carry *Borrelia* species including *Ixodes angustus, Ixodes banksi* (beaver tick), *Ixodes cooke*i (groundhog tick), *Ixodes gregsoni, Ixodes muris, Haemaphysalis leporispalustris* (rabbit tick), and *Dermacentor albipictus* (winter tick). *Rickettsia/Rocky Mountain Spotted Fever* is carried by the soft bodied *Dermacentor variabilis* tick and the Rocky Mountain wood tick *Dermacentor andersoni* (Peavey, et al., 2000).

Relapsing fever, as its name implies, is an illness characterized primarily by recurrent fevers. It is caused by at least fifteen species of the genus *Borrelia*. It can be vectored to humans by either lice or ticks. Lice-borne Relapsing Fever tends to occur in epidemic waves, usually at times of human crisis such as war, deep poverty and/or overcrowding. Epidemics followed both World War I and World War II in Europe, resulting in over a million deaths.

Tick-borne Relapsing Fever can be transmitted by soft-bodied ticks of the genus *Ornithodoros* that feed for short periods and tend to take their meals at night. Their bites are painless. Tick-borne relapsing fever is endemic primarily in Africa, Central Asia, the Mediterranean, Central and South America, and in western parts of the United States and southern British Columbia in Canada (Dworkin, et al., 2008).

Tularemia is a rare but serious infection caused by the bacterium *Francisella tularensis*. The microbe has been found in many species of mammals, birds, amphibians, arthropods, and even fish. The disease occurs throughout North American and Eurasia. In the United States, it is most prevalent in the western and south-central parts of the country. The main animal hosts are small mammals like rabbits and hares. They acquire the organism through the bite of an infected tick or by contact with contaminants in the environment. In humans, infection is usually caused by bites from *Dermacentor* or *Amblyomma* ticks in summer or through contact with rabbit carcasses in winter (Nigrovic & Wingerter, 2008).

Since Lyme disease was first discovered, named, and became recognized by the medical community, incidence rates have risen steadily on a world wide basis. This may reflect the fact that the disease is spreading, especially as the climate warms, but in reality it has been present for millions of years with ebbs and flows in prevalence and virulence. Climate and cultural practices all play a role in these rates.

Tick-borne infections are zoonotic—meaning that they are passed from animals to humans: in specific places, where tick survival is good, and during specific times of the year. The *Ixodes* tick is a crawling facilitator of pathogenesis via multiple infective agents. It can carry within its guts *Borrelia* and co-infections, all at the same time, and transmit them with a single bite. Lyme disease is found in the temperate deciduous forests of Europe, parts of China, Africa, Australia, North America and parts of South America-anywhere that is inhabited by *Ixodes* ticks or other possible vectors. The pan-endemic occurrence of Lyme disease is probably the strongest evidence to support a lengthy and protracted

history for the bacteria. One DNA sequencing study has led to a hypothesis that the *Borrelia* pathogen is distantly derivative from African Swine Fever, which has a similar relapsing life cycle, mammal host vector (warthogs), and arthropod (louse) mechanism for spreading (Hinnebusch and Barbour, 1991). It may have spread out of Africa along with migrating animals but existed even before the supercontinent of Pangaea broke apart.

In parts of Africa, there is a long history of *tick fever*, which is spread by mammal vector hosts (moles, rats and mice) and soft *Ornithodoros sonrai* ticks. After being eradicated in the 1950's, tick fever has re-emerged as a major public health threat in the northwestern African countries of Senegal, Mali and Mauritania due to the concentration of water seeking people, vector hosts, and vectors during a severe drought (Kaf-Ngoine, 2006).

Ixodes ticks are found in temperate forested regions with high relative humidity at ground level. In New England, *Ixodes scapularis* ticks thrive in sandy soil, deciduous forest and the edge habitats bordering forests that contain leaf litter. Moisture plays an important role in tick survival.The tick's need for both hydration and blood meals, as a matter of life or death, has led to the evolution of some exquisitely specialized sensory equipment.
Researchers have found that the tick's forelegs contain both organs that are sensitive to liquid water and a *different* set of organs that are sensitive to water vapor.

Ticks appear to avoid direct contact with water but need a certain level of humidity to maintain body torpor. The tick hydrates with a three-stage process. First, it uses its forelegs to detect micro-regions of high humidity, such as the area surrounding water droplets. Once a water source is detected, the tick salivates (spits) a hydrophilic solution from its barbed hypostome mouth. It can absorb moisture from air that is at a forty one percent or more humidity level. When this blob of saliva solution is saturated by water from the humid air, the tick draws it back into its mouth to drink. A tick also spits hydrophilic solution to absorb liquid during a blood meal. In this process it also expels pathogens from the gut into the blood meal host(Kröber & Guerin, 1999).

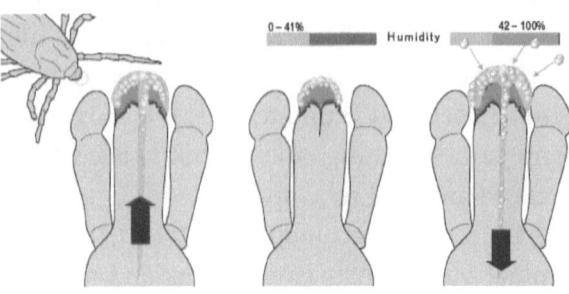

Figure 3. HOW TICKS ABSORB MOISTURE.www.asknature.com

The tick's salivary glands are the site where pathogens are harbored and the injection of a thick blob of saliva solution during feeding is the route for pathogen transmission. It is theorized that because blood is deficient in B vitamins, some bacteria may act as symbionts in tick digestion by adding missing nutrients through their waste processes (Bowman & Sauer, 2004).

Using its calcified barbed harpoon and straw like hypostome mouth to puncture skin, and palps to latch on and hold it in place, ticks first secret saliva that is infused with an anesthetic that numbs the attachment site, and then injects an anti-coagulant that thins blood before they drink it. When feeding, the tick's digestive system strains key nutrients from blood but then spits about seventy percent of the fluid and ion content of the blood back into the host. Tick saliva contains many bioactive protein and lipid components as well as infective pathogens. As they feed, ticks grow into plump blood filled spheres, and then fall off the host when satiated. It is during this process that *Borrelia* infection begins. *Ixodes scapularis* are small but can stretch in size when engorged with blood (Sauer, et al., 2000).

Tick attachment can cause tick paralysis, which results from exposure to a neurotoxin that is released by tick salivary glands during a blood meal; it is the only tick-borne disease not caused by an infectious agent. The toxin appears to be produced exclusively by female, egg-laden ticks. It is most commonly seen in children and adult males. Worldwide, over forty tick species have

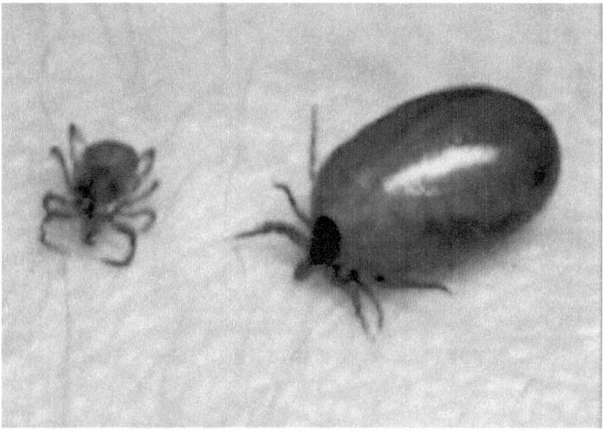

Figure 4. BEFORE AND AFTER A BLOOD MEAL.
www.mass.gov.

been associated with tick paralysis, but in America the most common culprits are *Dermacentor variabilis* and *Dermacentor andersoni*. Bites from *Amblyomma* and *Ixodes* ticks can also cause tick paralysis (Edlow, et al., 2008). *Ixodes* ticks are generally found within eight feet of the edge between heavily wooded areas and tracts of cleared land- the transitional ecotone that is also the favored habitat of mice and deer. In areas where most of the land has been cleared of trees, ticks may be limited to stone walls and shrubby riparian areas.

Knowing the complex life cycle of the *Ixodes* tick is important in understanding the risk for humans of acquiring Lyme disease and other tick-borne infections. The *Ixodes tick* has a two-year life cycle and three life stages. Adult female ticks lay eggs on the ground in early spring. By summer, the eggs will have hatched into larvae. Larvae feed on mice, small mammals, and birds in the late summer and early fall, and then they molt into nymphs that burrow into leaf litter, and are inactive until the next spring. Nymphs feed on rodents, small mammals, birds, and humans in the late spring and summer and then molt into adults by the fall. In the fall and spring, adults feed and mate on large mammals (usually deer) and can also attach to humans.

The key role that deer play in this cycle is that they can nourish a large number of ticks, assuring population viability and stability, and, move the ticks around from place to place. Where the deer are is geographically also where the ticks will be most heavily concentrated. However, deer do not contract or spread the Lyme bacteria. Deer have an antibody to the Outer Surface Proteins [Osp] of the spirochete in their blood (their health is usually not affected) which acts prophylactically to eliminate the bacteria in adult ticks during their last blood meal. *Ixodes* ticks use deer hosts as mating grounds. After mating, male adults drop off and die.

When an adult female drops off, she lays bacteria-free fertilized eggs, which completes her two-year life cycle. In the majority of cases, larvae hatch in an uninfected state and are only infected after contact with their first blood meal host. Ticks, birds, rodents, and some other animals all serve as natural reservoirs for the *Borrelial* spirochete, which live and grow within these hosts without causing death. Once infected, the tick remains infected for the rest of its' life- up until the final deer blood meal. Ticks search (quest) for blood meal hosts from the tips of grasses, shrubs, and leaf litter and transfer onto animals or people that brush against this vegetation. Ticks can only crawl. They do not fly or jump. Ticks cling to any part of the body but on a human they will most often crawl to a moist hidden area like the groin, armpit, or a place near the waist (Columbia University, 2017).

Like so many other features of any landscape, the prevalence of Lyme disease is directly influenced by both nature and the 'hand of man.' Glaciation has had a strong effect on the bacteria, the *Ixodes* tick vector, and humans down to a genetic basis. High prevalence rates for Lyme disease currently skirt northern latitudes, wherever there are deciduous mixed forests with enough leaf litter for ticks to stay hydrated. These forests are often located in geographic areas that were influenced by the most recent glaciation that ended 20-15,000 years ago. It has been observed that species diversity in many animals and plants decreases in northern latitudes (Anderson & Borns,1997).

In a North American genetic study of the *Ixodes scapularis*

tick, substantial differences have been found in the genetic structure and evolutionary history of the ticks that are found in northern areas when compared to ticks that are found in inland southern areas. Coastal areas are a blur of genes due to bird migration mixing the genetics up. For a while, there was a debate over whether both sets of ticks were even the same species. Although they are taxonomically now described as the single species, *Ixodes scapularis,* distinct differences have been identified within the species.

The population structure was separately analyzed using a subset of representative DNA Single Nucleotide Polymorphisms. Membership probabilities, interpreted as proximities of individuals belonging to each cluster, revealed five clades or family groupings for *Ixodes scapularis*. Indiana and New Hampshire cluster together, and the Massachusetts, Maine, and Wisconsin form a cluster, indicating significant shared alleles, while the Southern population in Virginia, Florida and North Carolina share only a small number of alleles, showing little spread (Gulia-Nuss, et al 2016).

In northern North America, where *Ixodes scapularis* populations feed predominantly on white-footed mice as nymphs and on deer as adults, Lyme disease is a clear and present danger. In contrast, southern populations exploit a wider range of vertebrate hosts and are not quiescent during winter. The variety in blood meal hosts available with their varying levels of *Borrelia* tolerance seems to dilute the prevalence of Lyme disease in the South.

The "American clades" (formerly called *Ixodes dammini)* are located in the north and midwest (and also occasionally shows up in the mixed genetics of coastal southern areas having been brought down by migrating birds). The American clades show genetic evidence of exponential increases in population size. This population explosion came after the period of extreme contraction or 'evolutionary bottleneck' caused by glaciation. Genetic patterns in southern populations show a long evolutionary history of constant and stable population size. The lower rate of *Borrelia burgdorferi* infection in southern *Ixodes scapularis* ticks could be the result of the more diverse genetic heterogeneity in southern ticks as well as the different levels of infected blood meal hosts (Goddard, et al. 2015).

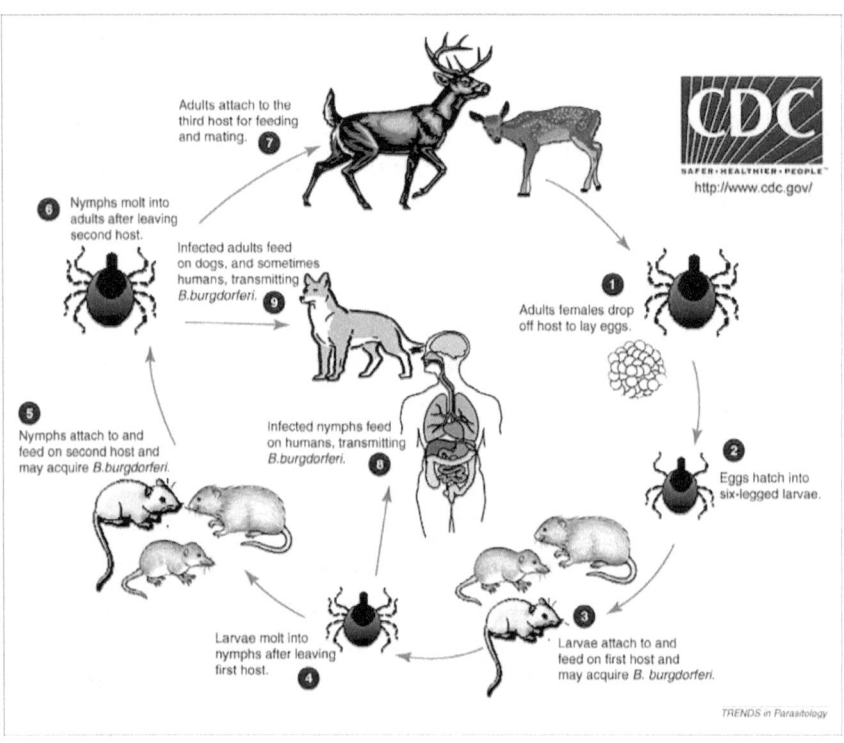

Figure 5. Schematic of the ecology of Lyme disease. The tick vector has three stages, larvae, nymphs and adults, which each take one blood meal (except adult males) before molting into the next stage or reproducing and dying (adult females). Adult female ticks feed primarily on deer, whereas the other two stages feed from a wide range of vertebrates including mammals, birds and reptiles with widely varying probabilities of infecting ticks. Host species are eaten by a suite of interacting predators, and their populations are influenced by fluctuations in food, like acorns, availability. CDC.

Ixodes ticks need an area with an optimum level of moisture to survive. The largest deciduous forests of the earth today are the result of re-growth after glaciation. A study of a forest/tundra ecotone in modern Colorado found that tree establishment is correlated with climate. The territory inhabited by humans, ticks, and *Borrelia* has changed: it contracted and expanded over time. In the past, the warming of the atmosphere after the glaciations of North America created a slowly moving set of transitional zones, or ecotones (Hessel &Baker, 1997).

At 18,000 years before the present (BP), for example, the modern state of Massachusetts was tundra at the edge of a glacier. This, in turn, edged a larger swath of conifer-dominated zones that covered most of the eastern seaboard, the Midwest, and the upper Southern geography. The humid temperate/conifer mixed woodland that would have been good *Ixodes* tick habitat was then restricted to two zones on either side of the Proto-Mississippi River on what is now the southern Gulf Coast. This correlates roughly with an area in Tennessee that archeologists have described as "The Cradle of Rheumatoid Arthritis" due to the amount of joint bone infection found in ancient human remains. It may actually be "The Cradle of Lyme Disease" for North America (Rothschild,et al.,1988).

One recent study has proposed the idea that ecotones are a source of flora and fauna speciation, which appears to have almost happened in North American tick populations. Pleistocene glaciation events have caused parallel biogeographic patterns of reduced genetic variability in the north for a wide range of other animal and plant species, including humans, on a worldwide basis. During Glaciation Maximums, most of Europe, much of North America, and parts of China were covered in ice. Human as well as tick populations found refuges from the cold and ice where they could (Delcourt & Delcourt,1992). It was in these refuges that the the foundations of many aspects of modern cultures and differentiated group genetic characteristics [haplogroups] and innate immune responses were formed. In Europe, populations were pushed south into havens on land that is now in Spain and Portugal, into the Middle East, and out onto an ice-clear patch

Table 1. CHART OF TICK AFFLICTED OVER TIME

Afflicted	When	Where[modern]	Affliction	Activity	Promote/Protect
Tick	100MYBP	[Myanmar]	Palaeorickettsia		
Primate	20MYBP	[Dominican Republic]	Babesia microti	Grooming	
Tick	15MYBP	[Dominican Republic]	Paleoborrelia		
Nandy	80KBP	Shalimar Cave[Iran]	Bone infections	Hunter/gatherers	Fire Use
Glacial Refugees China & Southern Europe	LGM	Ice free Temperate Forest	Bone infections	Hunter/gatherers	Fire Use
Cherokee, Creek, Tchefuncte	10KBP	Tennessee, Kentucky, Alabama, Ohio	Bone infections	Hunter/gatherers	Respect for sick deer, Fire Use
Yamnaya	8KBP	Central Asia to Northern Europe, India and Western China	—	Pastoral Herding	Trousers, grassland, Cannabis
Otzi	5KBP	Bolzano, Italy area	Borrelia	Shepherd/hunter	Fire Use, Antibiotic herbs, Acupuncture
Chickens	10KBP-2017	Southeast Asia/India-Egypt-worldwide	Borrelia anserinas		
Cats	12KBP-2017	Middle East/China-Egypt-Rome-Worldwide	Bartonella	catch mice	Decrease in mouse and rat populations
Yellow Emperor	2KBP	Yellow River, China	Spirochetal illness	traditional herbal medicine	herbal cures
Richard I	1157-1199AD	European travel, Holy Land	Borrelia vincenti TBRF-viral?	Crusading	Travel in tick-risky areas, poor hygiene, poor nutrition, crowded conditions
Witch Hunts	1450-1750 AD	Europe, N. America	Borrelia?	Living in rural environment Cat	Folklore
Catherine of Aragon	1485-1536 AD	England	Babesia?	The Hunt	Hunting contact with deer, long skirts,

M=million
K=thousand
BP=years before 1950
LGM=Last Glacial Maxima
AD=Anno domini, since 0, it is now 2017 AD.

that would became the grassy steppes of the modern Ukraine and Russia. The people who would eventually reach into the Americas were forced at first to inhabit zones in Asia, The Himalayan Mountains were glaciated and deciduous forest was constrained to a small coastal zone in what is modern China. Humans may have become incidental hosts for *Borrelia* and ticks that were also in refuge from the cold and ice in the same places (Anderson & Borns,1997).

Biodiversity plays a key role in the spread of Lyme disease. Where ticks have a wide variety of blood meal hosts they maintain a lower rate of *Borrelia burgdorferi* infection due to the variability of host transmission capacities for the bacteria. This is called the Dilution Effect Model. Lizards (especially in the south), opossums, and squirrels, for example, are poor *Borrelia burgdorferi carriers*. But, in reverse, when ticks feed on a limited number of species of animals that are good transmitters (white-footed mice and birds) there can be a dramatic rise in the level of infected ticks. The 'hand of man' has helped to decrease the number of species living in the world today. Certain species, like the passenger pigeon, have been hunted to extinction. Other species, like deer and beaver, tottered close to extinction and then rebounded in some areas (LoGiuudice, et al. 2003). Man has used fire to clear land [which kills ticks]since at least the Mesolithic Period (Innes & Blackford, 2003). Domesticated animals have also played a role by competing with indigenous animals for food and territorial space and as blood meal hosts for ticks.

Forested landscapes have been carved up and fragmented. The world's forests were extensively altered by early hunter/gatherer groups, deforested by herding and farming settlers, but, in many parts of the United States, Europe and Eurasia, have been reforested during the past one hundred and fifty years due to farm abandonment and industrialization. It is estimated, for example, that the forested areas of New England are now at a level of acreage equal to that extant during the Revolutionary War period (Foster & O'Keefe, 2000).

Two modern studies have found a relationship between forest fragmentation and disease. Research done at the University of

Florida found that fragmented forests had higher concentrations of parasites and that animals living within the fragments suffered from a higher level of infection than those living in undisturbed areas. This may be related to an almost unavoidable interaction with the stressors of an encircling edge environment (n.a.,2000, September). A study of birds in western Minnesota, for example, found that brood parasitism was higher in nests located near a wooded edge than those located far from an edge (Gustafson, 2002). Another study found that the density and infection rates for *Ixodes scapularis* ticks with Lyme disease was dramatically higher in small forest fragments. Fragments that totaled less than five acres carried a Lyme disease risk that was seven times greater than that found in larger areas. This was also found to correlate with a high population of white-footed mice in these same forest fragments (Allan, Keesing, & Ostfeld, 2003).

Like everything else involved with Lyme disease, explanations for the episodic and epidemic level of virulence among humans and ticks is complex and still subject to much study. Good tick habitat is not static. Modern scientists use several factors to predict the amount of risky 'tick friendly' habitat a geographic area contains. Tick densities are highest in moist but well drained areas with sandy soils over underlying sedimentary bedrock. Because the immature stages of *Ixodes* ticks require leaf litter to overwinter, they prefer a forest that includes deciduous trees that drop their leaves in the fall. The brushy transition zone under trees and between forest and cleared land is most likely to harbor questing ticks. In areas where land is open or grasslands, especially during droughts, tick populations are concentrated in river corridors (Guerre,et al., 2002).

Drought causes animals to move around in search of water. One study compared the number of mice found along a hiking path during a year of normal rainfall with the number found during a drought year. The number decreased from more than two hundred to two mice. It is theorized that the mice had either died or, more likely, simply moved to an area with higher moisture levels or access to water-somewhere near a river or lake. In fact riparian corridors, sandy soil, and wooded vegetation have been found to be

strongly correlated with clusters of *Ixodes* ticks and are Lyme disease foci. During droughts, tick presence on mice and deer is associated with proximity to rivers (Jones & Kitron, 2000). The drought of 1566 in England, for example, may have led to rodent and tick concentration near rivers. The prolonged drought suffered by the Massachusetts Bay Colony during the early 1690's may have had a similar concentrating effect on the mice and ticks along the Ipswich River.

The story of the history of Lyme *borreliosis* as an *old* disease would read something like the following: After the retreat of the ice at the end of the Last Glacial Maxima, the dynamics of climate, trees, mast [acorns and other tree nuts], deer, mice, birds, ticks, and bacteria continued and expanded in a long and intrinsically complicated set of interactions that still occur in modern times. For the most part, they take place across a swath of the earth's land surface- girdling the forty to fifty degree latitude marks in the northern hemisphere, wherever *Ixodes* ticks are known to thrive. Today this swath may be expanding due to global warming (Brownstein, et al., 2005).

When environmental conditions are just right, Lyme disease can become endemic, often in a dispersed, splotchy, localized, dynamic with edges that are also blurred by the movement of various species of animals and birds. Ticks that have ended up as museum specimens, going as far back as the 19th century and up to the 1940's on Long Island, New York, have been found to be infected with *Borrelia* (Pershing,et al. 1990, Matuschka, et al., 1996). In the middle of the Twentieth Century, moderns humans began to move into a landscape pattern that helped create today's pandemic of Lyme disease affliction.

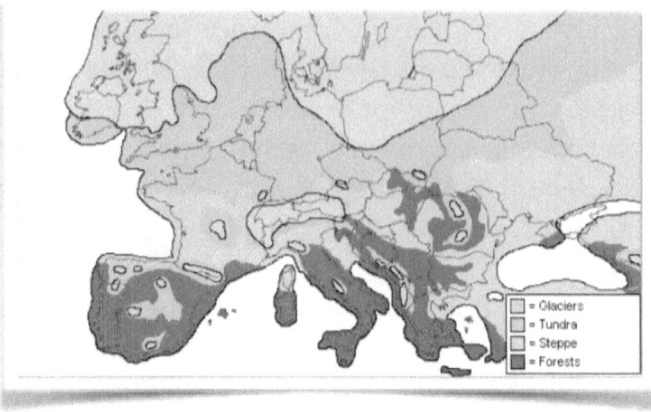

Europe

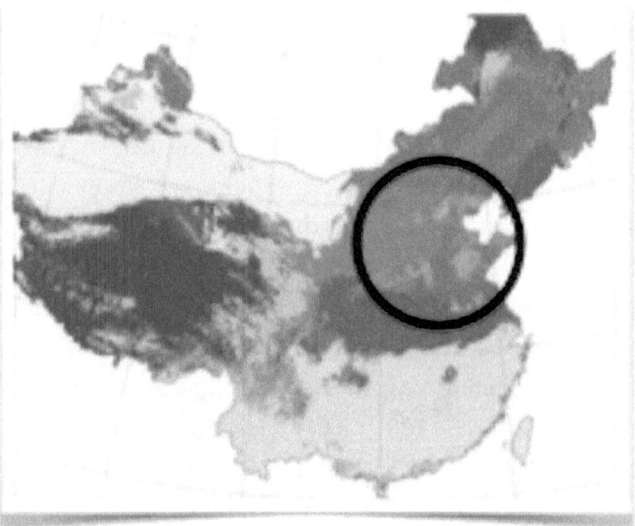

China

Figure 6. LAST GLACIAL MAXIMA. Glaciation caused the deciduous forest in Europe [top] to shrink down to the rim areas of The Mediterranean and around The Black Sea. In China it was mixed in one area. Over the past 10,000 years the Deciduous Forest and tick habitat has expanded. Broadleaf forest provides good habitat for *Ixodes* ticks. Refuge tick populations were restricted to parts of North America, small bits of southern Europe, and China during the Last Global Maxima(circled area). Humans found refuge from the ice. In Eurasia, isolated human populations found refuge in grassy steppe areas and forested zones. Cultures that were developing in what would become China thrived in less stark climatic conditions. As the climate warmed, temperate forests were re-positioned in the north, making those areas tick risky again.(American Geophysical Union, 2003, Wang, et al., 2017).

THE PERSISTENT SPIRAL

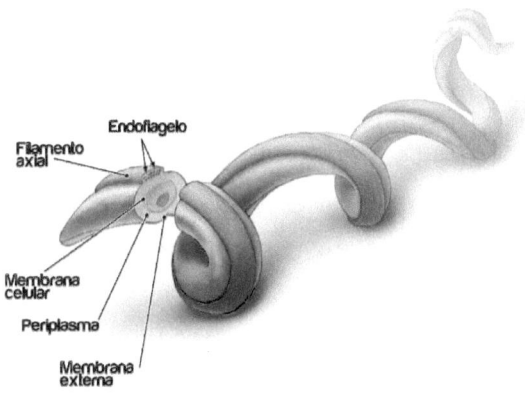

Figure 7. The structure of a Borrelia spirochete. Courtesy www.lyme.org.

The genus *Borrelia* is not closely related to any other bacteria and has a highly unusual genome composed of a linear chromosome with multiple circular and linear plasmids that appear to be in a constant state of rearrangement, recombination, and deletion. The determination of the genome sequence of *Borrelial* strains has facilitated an understanding of this genus at the molecular and cellular level, as well as the pathogenesis of the Lyme disease and relapsing fever that it causes (Radolf & Samuels, 2010, p.377).

Lyme disease risk is primarily dependent upon three factors within a landscape: the presence of *Ixodes* ticks, blood meal hosts for the ticks, and the presence of *Borrelia* bacteria and/or its co-infections. Lyme disease is caused by several types of the spiral shaped *Borrelia*: *Borrelia burgdorferi, Borrelia mayonii, Borrelia miyamotoi, Borrelia afzelii* and *Borrelia garinii*.

Borrelia burgdorferi and *Borrelia mayonii* cause Lyme disease in the United States, while *Borrelia afzelii* and *Borrelia garinii* are the leading causes of Lyme disease in Europe and Asia. *Borrelia turicatae* is a newly discovered species that infects dogs. There are probably more to be discovered. When the gene sequences of *Borrelia* flagellin were studied and compared, it was found that all strains share between 73.7 and 99.7 percent of genes (Fukanaga, 1996). *Paleoborrelia,* the ancestor of the modern bacteria, is over fifteen million years old (Poinar,2014). The modern *Borrelia burgdorferi* bacteria in North America has been traced by DNA sequencing back to a speciation event that occurred during the Paleolithic Era at more than 60,000 years ago. Lyme disease is endemic in temperate forests in North America, Northern Europe, China and Northern Asia, and Australia- anywhere that *Ixodes* ticks can find a good habitat.

The term 'Lyme disease' was first coined in 1975 by Dr. Allen Steere, a member of the United States Epidemic Intelligence Service, a branch of the United States Center for Disease Control[hereafter CDC]. Steere was sent to study a "cluster" of sick children who were living in the geographical area surrounding Old Lyme, Connecticut. They seemed to be suffering from an unusually high incidence rate of juvenile rheumatism. By 1977, Steere was announcing that he had discovered a new vector-borne disease that he named after the geographic epicenter of the newly discovered epidemic. Steele identified one symptom in some of these patients that appeared to be uniquely characteristic of the disease: the bull's-eye rash. While many people complained of other symptoms, Steere selected only those patients with bull's-eye rashes to participate in his initial seminal study. The causative spirochete was later discovered by Dr. Wily Burgdorfer in 1982, and appropriately named *Borrelia burgdorferi* (Murray, 1996).

Because of its importance as a pathogen and the value of complete genome sequence information for understanding its life cycle, the *Borrelia burgdorferi* bacteria was subjected to a gene sequencing study in the late 1990's. It was found to contain a linear chromosome of 910,724 base pairs. The most recent common ancestor of all *Borrelia burgdorferi* clades in North America most likely evolved in the Northeast coastal area.Virulence, based on $OSPc$ serotypes, is highest in the Northeast United States.The *Borrelia burgdorferi sensu stricto* clade has been found to have a complex evolutionary history with previously undocumented levels of migration. This diversity is ancient and geographically widespread, pre-dating the Last Glacial Maximum and the arrival of humans from Asia (Walter, et al., 2017). Pathogen genomes can reveal the history of epidemics. Phylogeography provides a

powerful framework for understanding pathogen evolutionary dynamics including probable epidemic origins, rates and patterns of spread, and the distribution of virulence.

A study of bacterial population variation, patterns of gene flow across North America, and the timescale of bacterial evolution has found that **all** available **European** *Borrelial* **genomes are related to each other and also to** a clade that is found in **American** Midwestern samples which suggests a complex pattern of genetic differentiation including bidirectional gene flow between regions (Fukunaga, et al.1996).

Scientists have found an observed substitution rate of 7.49×10^{-6} gene substitutions per site per year, which is faster than was previously estimated for *Borrelia burgdorferi*. This probably reflects the bacterium's ecology. When the spirochete is transmitted from tick to blood meal host to tick, its population experiences severe bottlenecks, so that only a fraction of the variants get transmitted to the next host. *Borrelia burgdorferi* diversity is ancient and long pre-dates not only the modern Lyme epidemic but also the Last Glacial Maximum (Walter, et al, 2017).

On a worldwide basis, current Lyme disease foci are in regions once covered by the Pleistocene ice sheets. Refugia for many animals, including humans, were located in southern areas and, after glacial retreat, southern migrants re-colonized the north. The ancient timescale of *Borrelia burgdorferi* diversification in North America suggests that this species was endemic in North America and Europe before the Pleistocene glaciation and its evolutionary history was shaped by ancient geological events that pre-date the ongoing modern Lyme epidemic.

Borrelia burgdorferi genomes change through the recombination of short genomic tracts along the chromosome and plasmids and by shuffling the shape of entire plasmids through recombination. Recombination hotspots include the major antigen O*spC*, *dbpA* and *dbpB*. These surface-expressed antigens experience selection imposed by host immune responses. The bacteria spreads through the movement of its vertebrate hosts like small mammals and birds. Instead of finding strong barriers to

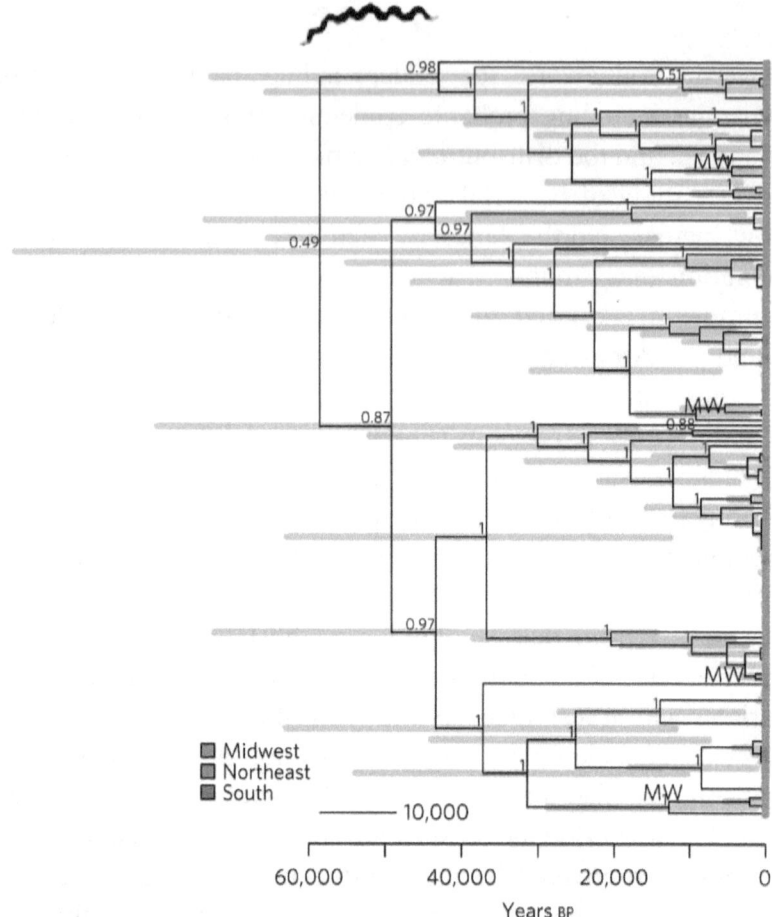

Figure 8. AN OLD PATHOGEN-Maximum Clade Credibility tree of the best-fitting model inferred with BEAST (relaxed log-normal molecular clock model; Bayesian skyline population size) for *Borrelia burgdorferi ss* in North America shows deep history. Evidence of ancient midwestern ancestry (the oldest internal node in each clade with support for ancestral location in the midwest) is labelled 'MW'. Branch lengths are in years BP, showing that Borrelia burgdorferi ss existed in North America for over 100,000 years, even before human migrants arrived. Branches are labelled with posterior probability values (not shown for shallow nodes for clarity). Dated phylogeny of *B. burgdorferi* in North America from information in Walter, et al, 2017.

gene flow between geographic areas, evidence of long-distance migration events due to long-distance dispersal have been found.

Dispersal by small mammals probably also contributes to gene flow on much smaller spatial scales. *Borrelia burgdorferi* infection often lags behind tick invasion, which means that epidemiological surveillance should focus on areas that have established *Ixodes* tick populations because they are potential sites for introduction of Lyme disease (Ostfeld & Brunner, 2015).

Lyme has been causing bone infections and Lyme arthritis in humans for eons. Ötzi, who lived five thousand years ago had *Borrelia* deep within his bones. An individual's response to *Borrelia* infection has genetic roots. Antibiotic-refractory Lyme arthritis has been found to be strongly associated with specific alleles or haplotypes, especially with various Major Histocompatibility Complex versions of Human Leukocyte Antigens [HLA]DR and DQ, part of the adaptive immune system (Kovalchuka,et al, 2015).

A study that compared joint damage in skeletal populations dating from between 7000 years BP to 400 years BP has found that Hunter-Gatherers, who frequently interacted with tick risky forest edge areas in pursuit of game, suffered from a higher rate of arthritis of the knees than Agriculturalists, who lived in relatively modified and tick-free zones, especially when they used fire as a landscape modifier (Inoue, et al, 2001). Another study found that arthritis of the knee was higher in pre-historic than early industrial populations but that post-industrial modern suburbanites have shown a dramatic surge in knee infection and arthritis since the middle of the twentieth century (Wallace,et al., 2017). When coupled with a study showing measurably levels of spirochetes found in a 7000 year old Mesolithic European genome, the evidence for Lyme Disease persistence seems clear (Olade,et al., 2014).

Over time all *Borrelia* bacteria have developed a complex, shape shifting physiology with mechanisms to evade various host immune systems, to survive, and sometimes thrive. The spirochete rotates its flagella within its outer skin which causes a traveling wave of undulation of the entire body. It can physically screw its

spiral shaped self within protected tissue sites. And this spiral, in turn, has developed a full set of survival skills to keep from being destroyed by any host's immune system. When its movements were recently clocked by scientists they were found to be the fastest ever recorded for any spirochete, moving at a rate that is two orders of magnitude faster than the fastest moving human body cell. This "alacrity" in an organism that has bi- motor capacity, scientists have concluded, may well contribute to difficulties in spirochete clearance (Dever, et al., 1993). Response cells involved in the human immune system may not be fast enough to grab it!

In addition to speed, the bacterium is a shape shifter. Drop a Lyme spirochete into a vial of distilled water and it will transform itself. The spirochete can develop a tough cyst to encase and protect the vital genetic material within its structure that it needs to replicate. These cysts are called persisters (Brorson,1998). The spirochetes can cluster together and form protective biofilms (Sapi,et al, 2012). In the blood stream of a host animal, the spirochetes sometimes sacrifice pieces of its casing proteins- spitting them off bits of various Outer Surface Proteins [OSP's] in a process called blebbing, which fools the immune system into uselessly chasing those bits of its former self around, while the now cell wall deficient form of the spirochete to safety within the host's own cell walls for protection. And there it can wait- sometimes for years- before it ever reverts to a spirochetes form again (Whitmire & Garon, 1993).

This may happen when the host is re-infected or when the immune system is weakened by things like co-infections, stress, sickness,accidents, nutrient deficiency, or the accumulated affects of aging. This may be one of the problems discovered during the Lymerix vaccine test trials- people who had a pre-existing inactive cyst form of the bacteria within their bodies found it transformed into an active spirochete infection by the injection of the new outer surface protein factor that the vaccine was made from, making them symptomatic. In some people with a genetic sensitivity, the inoculated outer surface proteins in the vaccine may have triggered an overzealous immune response that caused damage to

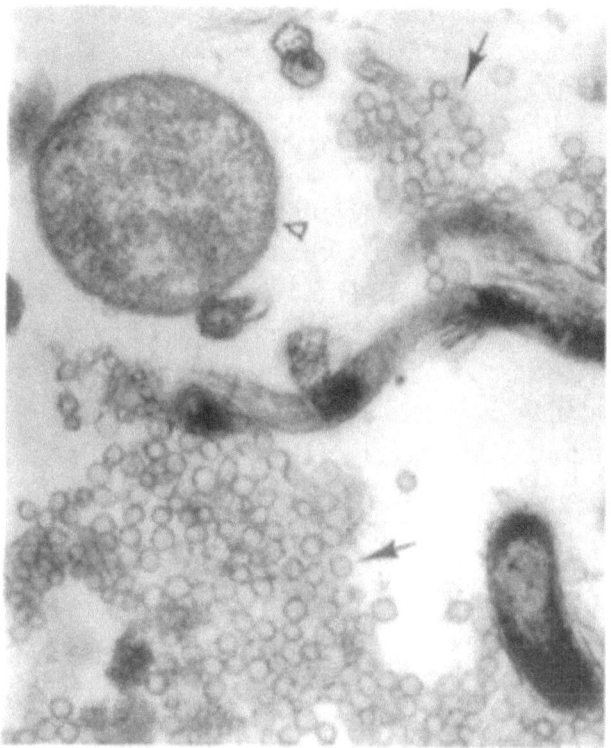

Figure 9. Electron photomicrograph of a thin section of *Borrelia hermsii* spirochetes exposed to benzylpenicillin for 10 hours. The spirochetes have turned into cysted persisters. An open triangle points to one example. Arrows indicate small membranous blebs of OSPs.
www.ncbi.nlm.nih.gov.

joints. Researchers have also found that the B*orrelia* bacterium contains aglycolipid that triggers an immune response from the body's natural killer T cells (lymenet.org).

The remarkable engineering of these bacteria is probably a major reason spirochetes have been such successful pathogens. Spirochetes are better at penetrating human bodies than almost any other organisms. Spirochetes cross barriers that are impenetrable to almost anything else. In humans, *Borrelia* easily penetrate the normally sacrosanct blood-brain barrier to infect the central nervous system. This extraordinary ability is reflected in the symptoms of this brutal disease. The characteristic Bullseye rash of Lyme disease seems to be the result of this penetrative ability, as the spirochetes burrow into the skin and soft tissue of their new host they trigger a destructive inflammatory response radiating from the bite that delivered them. Both Lyme Disease and syphilis sufferers, the latter of which have been legion among the great and small in human history, may experience damage to multiple organs, joints, and the brain and nervous system as a result damaging inflammation (Harman, et al 2013).

But there also appears to be a co-existing issue of *Borrelia* causing immunosuppression in some individuals. This mechanism may underlay cases of Chronic Lyme that present with a wide variety of symptoms: with a suppressed immune system whatever pre-existing bacterial, fungal, or viral infections that a patient carries within them that had been held at bay by a healthy immune system become free to wreak whatever variety of havoc they are capable of producing.

Humans, and the domesticated animals that they have become closely associated with, enter the Lyme disease picture when they become incidental blood meal hosts for *Ixodes* ticks. Unlike *Borrelia* and *Ixodes* ticks, which have spent millions of years evolving in earth's temperate forests, humans evolved as children of the grasslands. Having left the forest, humans carry within them a hybrid inherited innate immune system that produces a variety of results when infected with tick-borne pathogens.

Asymptomatic Lyme disease infections are somewhat

common. It should be emphasized that only a portion of those who ever test seropositive have symptoms and that the symptomatic can be seronegative, so this is still a confused and murky picture. Seropositivity can start at birth. One study of obstetrical patients and their infants in Lyme disease endemic areas found that eight percent of all newborns had cord blood that tested positive for Lyme antibodies (Silver,1997). Another study of infants born in endemic areas of New York State tested at a cord blood level of 10.2 percent seropositivity (Rahn,1991).

The seropositivity rate for domesticated animals in endemic areas has also been studied. Cows can become affected and calves can be born seropositive (Popvic, et al, 1993). Pigs, especially wild boar, have been found to harbor voluminous numbers of ticks and carry *Borrelia* but to date no research has been done on their role in the ecology of Lyme disease. In historic times, pigs were ubiquitous creatures of the woods but are generally absent from the oak forests of modern times (Greiner,et al.,1984). Dogs are prone to infection. One study found that seventy-five percent of all dogs in one area of Connecticut were seropositive, but of these, only five percent were symptomatic (Magnarelli, 1985). Another study found thirty-six percent of all cats in another town in Connecticut to be seropositive, again with only a few showing symptoms. There is considerable variation on a worldwide basis (Gibson, et al, 1993).

Based on these world-wide and history spanning studies of both humans and animals, and considering the lack of reliability of any of the current blood tests being used, Lyme infection should be looked at as a historic, pandemic, and omnipresent force. Some form of *Borrelia* were highly likely, at any point in historic time, to infect a percentage of all the people and animals in any possible endemic area. A percentage of them would become symptomatic for a variety of reasons. This would ebb and flow through time in response to changing environmental and cultural practices within various human societies, as well as varying bacterial loads, genetic sensitivities and technical changes like the use of fire, antibiotics, and vaccinations. Lyme disease appears in a variety of ways:

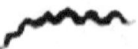

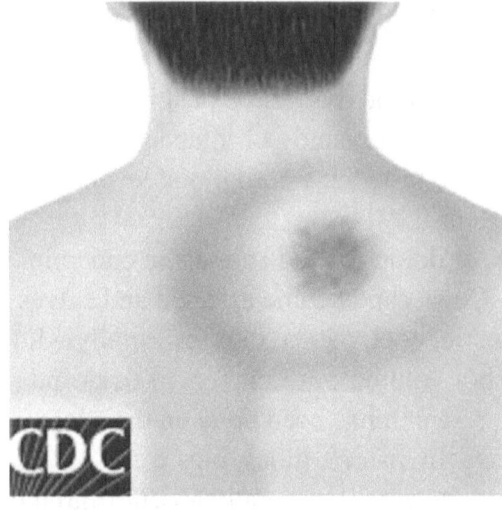

Figure 10. Bull's Eye Rash- Erythema Migrans.

1. as an acute infection with symptoms,
2. as a non-symptomatic infection,
3. in concert with one or more co-infections, and,
4. as chronic Lyme disease.

B*orrelia* and co-infections create a variety of symptoms and its virulence can vary from year to year and from person to person. Lyme disease is usually transmitted by the bite of a nymphal *Ixodes* tick in the spring and summer months or the bite of an adult in the late summer. Some infected persons will develop an Erythema Migrans (EM), also called a Bull's-Eye Rash, for obvious reasons. It begins at the site of the tick bite after a delay of between three to thirty days (average is about 7 days). The rash expands gradually over time and can reach up to twelve inches or more across. The rash may feel warm to the touch but is rarely itchy or painful. Sometimes a clear ring develops as it enlarges, resulting in a target-like appearance but can also appear as a range of rashes. An EM may be shaped like a ring, a triangle, an oval or even a long thin ragged line. The bulls-eye rash can re-occur throughout an infection.

Within days to weeks after the onset of local infection, pathogens may begin to spread through the body. Rashes may develop at sites across the body that bear no relationship to the original tick bite. It may cause inflammation in various joints. Various acute neurological problems, called neuroborreliosis, appear in ten to fifteen percent of untreated people.

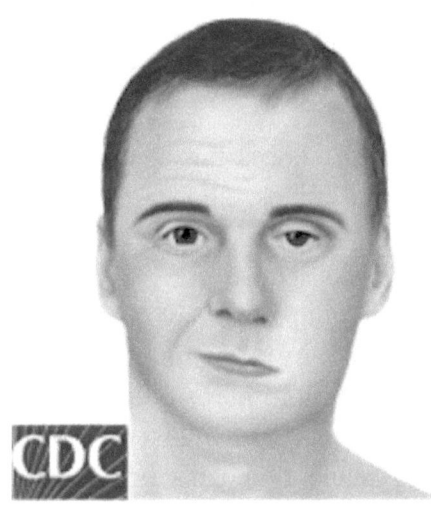

Figure 11. Bell's Palsy.

These include Bell's Palsy, which is the loss of muscle tone on one or both sides of the face, as well as meningitis, which involves severe headaches, stiff neck, and sensitivity to light. Seizures occur. After several months, some untreated or inadequately treated patients may go on to develop a late disseminated infection: severe and chronic symptoms that affect many parts of the body, including the brain, nerves, eyes, joints, and heart. The associated nerve pain radiating out from the spine is termed Bannwarth syndrome. This late disseminated stage is where the infection has fully spread throughout the body.

Chronic neurologic symptoms occur in some patients. They experience shooting pains, numbness, and tingling in the hands or feet. A neurologic syndrome called Lyme encephalopathy is associated with subtle cognitive difficulties, insomnia, a general sense of feeling unwell, and changes in personality. Chronic

encephalomyelitis, which may be progressive, can involve cognitive impairment, brain fog, migraines, balance issues, weakness in the legs, awkward gait, bladder problems, vertigo, and back pain.

In rare cases, Lyme disease can cause frank psychosis, which is misdiagnosed as schizophrenia or bipolar disorder. Panic attacks and anxiety can occur. Delusional behavior may be seen, including somatoform delusions, sometimes accompanied by a depersonalization or derealization syndrome, where the patients begin to feel detached from themselves or from reality (Drymon, 2008).

Lyme arthritis usually affects the knees but again, arthritis can occur in other joints, including the ankles, elbows, wrists, hips, and shoulders. Pain is often mild or moderate, usually with swelling at the involved joint. Baker's cysts may form and rupture. Joint erosion occurs. These arthritic symptoms may take a longer time to manifest. *Borrelia* have the ability to erode collagen and invade, colonize, and infect bones-adding to porosity and creating lesions. This is an important aspect of Lyme disease for the historian because most surviving ancient remains are found in skeletal form.

The presence of other tick borne co-infections add to or amplify the myriad array of Lyme symptoms. *Babesia* is a malaria-like parasite called a "piroplasm" that infects red blood cells. Under a microscope, infected red blood cells can sometimes look like they have been imprinted with a maltese cross. Victor Babes first identified this infective agent in 1888. *Babesia bigamina,* spread by the *Boophilis annulatus* tick, is the species that caused Texas Cattle Fever, a disease which nearly decimated the American cattle industry in the late nineteenth century. Research into that epidemic by the U.S.Department of Agriculture found that the disease had arrived in North America in the 1600s within cattle imported from the Spanish colonies of the West Indies and Mexico.

Babesia microti, the most common species infecting humans, was first identified in 1957. *Babesia* can also be transmitted from mother to unborn child or through blood transfusions. Symptoms

are similar to those of Lyme disease but babesiosis more often starts with a high fever and chills. The hallmark of *Babesia* is **drenching sweat**. As the infection progresses, patients may develop fatigue, headache, muscle aches, chest pain, hip pain and shortness of breath ("air hunger"). Complications include very low blood pressure, liver problems, severe hemolytic anemia (a breakdown of red blood cells), and kidney failure. The first modern case of human babesiosis was identified on Nantucket Island, Massachusetts, in 1969 (Krause & Feder, 1994).

Tick borne *Ehrlichiosis* is a term that was used for several different bacterial diseases which are now called *Anaplasmosis*. Some are transmitted by *Ixodes* ticks and others by the *Lone Star* tick. Its clinical manifestations are characterized by sudden high fever, fatigue, muscle aches, and headache. The disease can be mild or life-threatening. Severely ill patients have low white blood cell count, low platelet count, anemia, elevated liver enzymes, kidney failure and respiratory insufficiency. Death can occur (CDC).

Powassan virus can infect the central nervous system and cause encephalitis and meningitis. Symptoms can include fever, headache, vomiting, weakness, confusion, loss of coordination, speech difficulties, and seizures. Approximately half of survivors have permanent neurological symptoms, including recurrent headaches, muscle wasting and memory problems. Despite treatment approximately ten precent of this viral encephalitis cases are fatal (http://www.health.state.mn.us).

Additionally, evidence is growing for *Bartonella* as another tick-borne co-infection. Bartonella infects the inside lining of blood vessels. It can infect humans and a wide range of animals. *Bartonella henselae* was first 'identified' in 1990. It may have been spread around the world by cat domestication. It is transmitted to humans by fleas, body lice, and/or ticks. A recent study suggests that *Bartonella* can be passed from mother to unborn child. Scientists have identified several species of *Bartonella* on a worldwide basis. Early signs of *Bartonella* infection include fever, fatigue, headache, poor appetite, later symptoms include blurred vision, numbness in the extremities, memory loss, balance problems, headaches, ataxia (unsteady gait), and tremors. It is accompanied by an unusual streaked rash that resembles large scratches. Swollen glands are typical, especially around the head, neck and arms. Patients sometimes report a burning sensation on the soles of their feet and palms of their hands. *Bartonellosis* can trigger psychiatric manifestations and patients are more likely to have visited a neurologist than members of the general population (Schaller, 2008).

Rickettsia/Rocky Mountain Spotted Fever's may be related to Lyme disease in as yet unknown ways. When he was searching for the causative agent for Lyme Disease in 1981, Dr, Wily Burgdorfer found that Lyme patient blood samples also reacted strongly to the "Swiss Agent," identified as *Rickettsia helvetica* (Piller, 2016).

The activation of the dormant herpes *Epstein Barr Virus* after a Lyme infection can be accompanied by severe fatigue. *Mycoplasma* activation can also cause fatigue, respiratory problems, the sensation of chest pressure like a band around chest, and sometimes, increased salivation (CDC). This may have afflicted Andrew Jackson.

What would trigger the symptoms of Lyme disease and who would display them in the past? Using the logic that a portion of the population,especially while: 1. **interacting with an endemic area where** *Ixodes* ticks had found amenable habitat [usually deciduous forest edge with leaf litter] and *Borrelia* will be present at any point in historic time. Where did they live? Did they interact with the forest? Did they have contact with animals that might transfer ticks? The triggers for infection might be 2. **stress** of some sort: environmental[drought, famine,flooding], emotional, disease, social and/or physical change. 3. Certain **cultural activities and practices** would tend to either deter or promote infection. Activities like leaf burning, wearing protective clothing styles, the medicinal use of antibiotic substances, forest avoidance, and interactions with a diverse variety of animals might diminish spread of infection. Landscape neglect during warfare, contact with the forest during deforestation, the use of fire, camping, hunting, and other activities might facilitate infection. 4.**Tick populations** would be affected by masting, moisture levels, the movement of

blood meal hosts, and other environmental conditions. 5.**When would people show symptoms?** Ticks are present year round but most active during warm weather.This seasonality has been graphed for modern *Ixodes scapularis* populations. Most of the early symptoms of infection in the historic past would probably have also occurred at the times of year immediately following the peak periods (see below) for nymphal and adult tick activity. Arthritic and neurological symptoms could appear at any point in time. 6. **Who would show symptoms in the past?** Modern statistical studies in the United States have found that symptomatic cases of Lyme disease tend to be bimodal-affecting the young, especially males that are less than 14 years old, more heavily with another peak later in the age span in the older age groups. This pattern has been duplicated in various European studies. Throughout time and across cultures, children may tend to be inherently attracted to play in edge environments that are tick risky and may receive more ticks bites. A young immune system may also be more sensitive to infection, which creates the early incidence peak on the graph. 7. **Were people protecting themselves? Knowingly or unknowingly,** people who dressed protectively, wearing leather and thick fabrics, long sleeves, and trousers that were tucked into their socks would show fewer infections. People who employed insecticides and repellents would also have fewer symptoms. People who avoided the outdoors would have fewer infective opportunities.

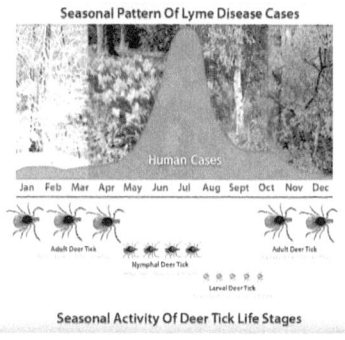

Figure 12. TickEncounter.org.

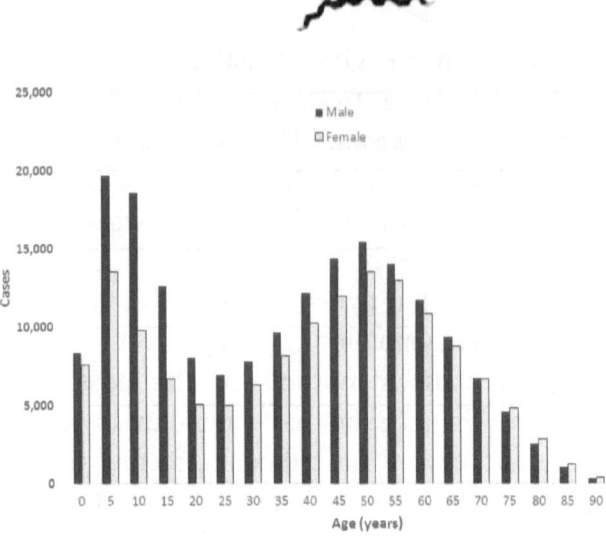

Figure 13. Distribution of Age and Sex- Lyme Disease Cases USA 2001-2015. The young and middle aged represent peaks.   CDC.

Modern research has found that because so many body systems are involved, Lyme disease can take on a wide array of forms. People with mild infections may show no signs at all. In other people, Lyme disease is so severe that it completely disrupts normal life. Lyme disease can become chronic, or it can follow a cyclical pattern of active infection, remission, and relapse. Except for fatigue and lethargy, which are often constant, the signs of Lyme disease are typified by their intermittent and changing nature. Lyme meningitis is often accompanied by irritability, photophobia, and impaired concentration. Neurological abnormalities may last for months but will usually resolve completely even without antibiotic therapy.

Lyme disease can infect the brain. The relatively recent development of brain scans, especially the MRI and SPECT technologies has made the brain damage done by *Borrelia* spirochetes visible to researchers for the first time. In neurological Lyme disease MRI scans have found white matter hyper-intensities in the brains of approximately fifteen to forty five percent of patients. These seem to be similar to the damage seen in multiple sclerosis patients (Agarwal &Sze, 2009).

Past human populations would probably have little concern for the *Ixodes* ticks that in their nymphal stage are only a little bigger than the period at the end of this sentence. They would probably have been virtually unaware of their presence in their environment. Attached adult ticks might have been noticed but not recognized as attached ticks. People were less likely to change clothing or do skin inspections in times when hygiene did not include much in the way of bathing. Rashes could have come and gone without much notice. After all, it took modern science several years to figure out the tick-bacteria-affliction connection and that research is still very much a work in progress. The "germ theory of disease" was in its infancy until the seventeenth century. But the advanced afflictions caused by the invisible world of bacteria would have been difficult to ignore.

The experience of Lyme disease can be understood by looking at the medical and scientific literature but it is also a very idiosyncratic condition that can only be described by the person experiencing the symptom or by an observer of the afflicted. Modern source material can be found that includes descriptions of the experiences of people with Lyme disease that can be compared to historic descriptions of human lives.

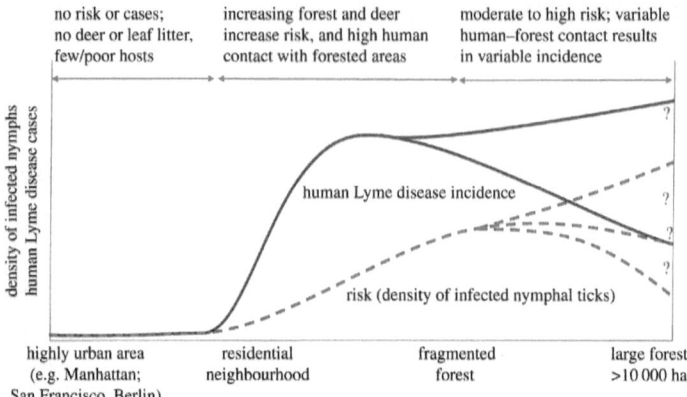

Figure 14. Landscape patterns of Lyme disease risk (density of infected nymphal ticks) and human incidence across a fragmentation gradient from highly urban areas (far left) to large forested areas (right) based on the available literature (see text). The mechanisms underlying the trends in both risk and incidence are given above the graph. The two blue and three red curves ending with question marks illustrate the variability and uncertainty in the pattern of incidence and disease risk in large forested areas. From Kilpatrick, et al, 2017.

Factors Associated With Risk for Lyme disease and Its Associated Manifestations

Predisposing Factors	Precipitating Factors	Perpetuating Factors
HLA DR2, HLA DR 4 TLR Genotype/Haplotype	Tick bite (initial infection)	High bacterial load
	Episode of acute stress (relapse)	Re- infection
Epigenetics of ancestors	stress	Misdiagnosis
Compromised immune System	PTSD (relapse)	Sleep deprivation
Infections that cause Immunosuppression	Immunosuppression (relapse)	Co-infections
Interaction with ecosystem that fosters Tick-borne disease (infection)	Vaccination (relapse)	Chronic un-remitting pain
Bb Osp C genotype- degree of pathogenicity	Co-infection (relapse)	Accident
		Corticosteroid Usage
Sunlight levels: Vitamin D levels deficiency	Vitamin D deficiency	Vitamin D
Outdoor activities/ lifestyle (infection)	Childbirth (relapse)	

Pre-Infection: Epstein Barr, mycoplasma, influenza, etc.
Based upon Treatment Guidelines for Lyme, Dr. Joseph Burrascano, Jr, 2008.

Table 2. *Some of these characteristics can be looked for in the past.*

QUESTIONING THE PAST:

1. Did anyone interact with a potential endemic area for Lyme disease? Where did they live?
2. Were they under stress?
3. Were cultural practices conducive to infection?
4. Were environmental conditions conducive to sustaining tick populations?
5. When did they show symptoms?
6. Who were they, is genotype available, did they have an experienced innate immune system?
7. Were they protecting themselves from tick attachment, knowingly or unknowingly. How did they dress?

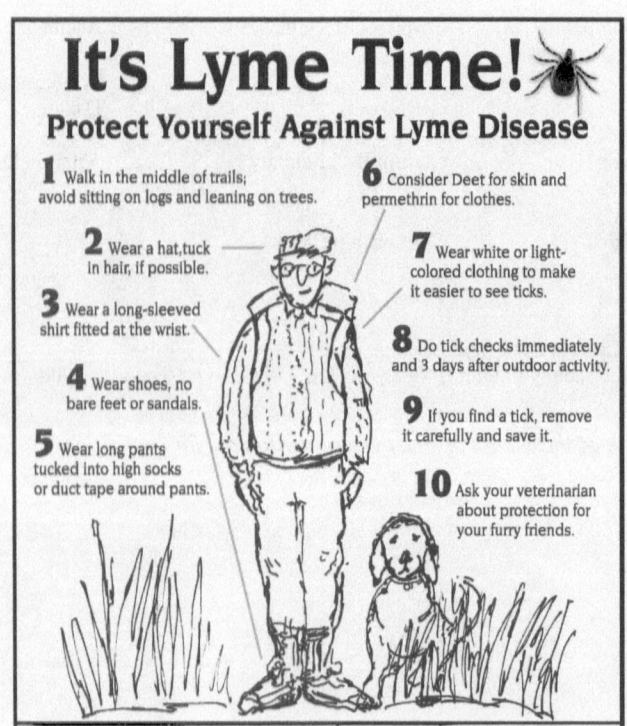

Figure 15. Modern Protection Recommendations. www.michigan.gov.

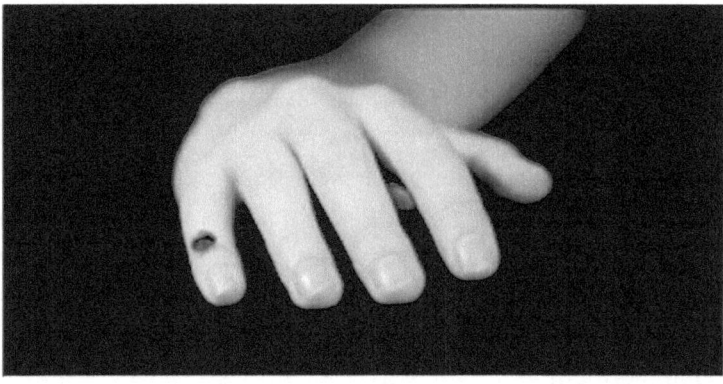

Figure 16. Replica of the analyzed bone fragment from a Denisovan that was used for DNA analysis, positioned on a living hand. Credit: Max Planck Institute for Evolutionary Anthropology.

IMMUNITY HAS ANCIENT ROOTS

As a species, we humans have confronted a daunting list of pathogens over time. Our immune system has developed and been trained by experiencing infection. All human immune systems differ from person to person and from place to place, dependent on the varying disease experiences of generations of past ancestors. In addition, each human's life experiences get added in, in the form of individualized adaptive immune systems.

Recent advances in genetic research have begun to rewrite the history of human interactions with pathogens. Prior to the understanding of DNA, a prevailing hypothesis had been that infectious disease had been low within the small groups of hunter/gatherers but skyrocketed with the spread of the Agricultural Revolution. By concentrating humans and animals together, it was theorized, pathogens made flying leaps from being the disease of domesticated animals into human afflictions. This was applied to explain influenza, smallpox, and measles (Furuse, 2010). Over time, the humans who domesticated big mammals were thought to have quickly built up immunities, because within each generation the individuals with better immunities had better chances of

survival to an age to reproduce.

Recent research has turned these ideas on their head. It turns out that many infectious diseases were instead tens of thousands of years older than previously thought and it was often the humans that infected the animals. After in-depth research, it was found that herd animals had become infected with tuberculosis only after they came into consistent contact with humans via domestication. Wild animals also seem to have acquired some of the pathogens that were brought out of Africa by migrating humans as well as the assemblage of bacteria, parasites, and companion species that accompanied them along the way(Latham, 2013).

Borrelia burgdoferi has ancestors that are millions of years old (Poinar, 2008). The *Borrelia* spirochete itself emerged during the Paleolithic Era and have been sporadically infecting humans ever since. The study of its DNA suggests that the pathogen has a complex history.The bacteria carry their genetic material in the form of a single, circular DNA molecule and in a segmented linear genome. Its chromosomes have closed endings called telomeres [a region of repetitive nucleotide sequences at each end of a chromosome which protects the end from deterioration or fusion with neighboring chromosomes] that are characterized by short hairpin loops of DNA. *Borrelia burgdorferi* carries three distinct subfamilies of Bdr [Borrelia direct repeat] proteins which suggests that there has been selective pressure to maintain multiple Bdr alleles and Bdr genetic diversity. This genetic diversity may have helped increase survival rates for the spirochete.

The Relapsing Fever spirochete species (*Borrelia parkeri* and *Borrelia hermsii*) are similar to Lyme disease (*Borrelia burgdoferi*) in that they carry Bdr genes on both linear and circular plasmids. Scientists have noted sequence similarities with poxviruses- particularly with the iridovirus agent of African swine fever. These findings suggest that the novel linear plasmids of *Borrelia* may have originated from a horizontal genetic transfer with a virus. It is possible that at some point in *Borrelia's* development it shared space with an iridopoxvirus inside soft bodied ancestral ticks before later switching to specialize in a symbiotic relationship with the hard bodied *Ixodes tick*.

Borrelia burgdorferi was the first bacterium for which linear plasmids and a linear chromosome were reported (Barbour & Garon, 1987, Baril et al.,1989, Ferrous & Barbour,1989). The genome of *Borrelia burgdorferi* is segmented and consists of a linear chromosome as well as at least 12 linear replicons that possess closed hairpin ends with near perfect inverted repeats at the telomeres (Hinnebusch & Tilly, 1993, Casjens et al., 1997, Casjens, 1999). Linear DNA with hairpin telomeres has also been reported in a diversity of other organisms including poxviruses, *Chlorella* virus, yeast mitochondrial plasmids, and *Escherichia coli* (Hinnebusch & Tilly, 1993; Casjens, 1999). In the case of *Borrelia*, the linear plasmid carries an Outer Surface Protein diversity generating system in which genetic information is moved onto an expression site that is adjacent to a telomere. It seems possible that these bacteria use the re-combinogenic properties of the ends of linear DNA molecules to augment this process (Casjens, 1999).

The iridopoxvirus *African swine fever* (ASFV) has hairpin telomeres that are similar in sequence to those located on *Borrelia*. If a linear ASFV-like chromosome had become integrated into the *Borrelia* ancestor's circular chromosome, it brought with it hairpin shaped telomeres and might have generated a linear molecule that could replicate in bacteria. This scenario is plausible because both *Borrelia* and ASFV are known to infect and are transmitted by arthropods.

The African *Ornithodoros* tick is photophobic and infests warthog burrows, where it finds a constant temperature and enough humidity to stay hydrated. In fact the African *Ornithodoros moubata* tick is known to transmit both *Borrelia duttoni* and ASFV, so it is reasonable that the genes of these two very distant and ancient biological phyla could have come into close contact and shared genetic material (Hinnebusch & Barbour,1991).

The history of migratory events and the changes in microbial populations which have led to the current species distribution on earth has been studied using phylogeographic tools incorporating geographic, ecological, and environmental correlates onto sequence-based phylogenies to address hypotheses and

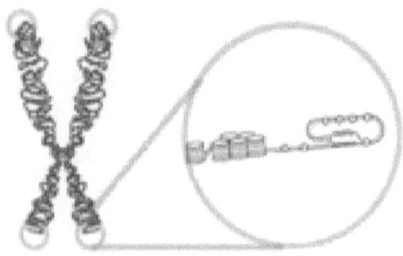

Telomeres are composed of coils of DNA. In *Borrelia,* they form a hairpin shaped ending. Chromosome pairs are located within a cell's nucleus.

Figure 17. A CHROMOSOME PAIR with hairpin telomeres.

interpret the patterns found in present day species distributions in light of historical events. Phytogeographic analyses of multiple loci for *Borrelia burgdorferi* sampled across a large geographic range produced an inferred migratory history of *Borrelia.* Evidence of limited historical gene flow suggested that in North America, past migration events originated in Eastern America and subsequently colonized the American Midwest . However, phylogenetic analyses of multiple loci have not resolved the debate on the geographic origin of *Borrelia* (Seifert, et al., 2015).

Different people react very differently to an infection with *Borrelia burgdorferi*. Age, environmental interactions, and genetic disposition all play important roles in disease progression. The *Borrelia* bacterium has a clear effect on the immune system. Variation in immune response can be largely explained by differences in the production of cytokines, the most important signaling molecules in the immune system. Lyme arthritis is associated with dysregulation of the [CD4] Cluster of Differentiation 4, T helper cells, and with some HLA-DR alleles. Cytokine production during a *Borrelia* infection was studied in five hundred healthy volunteers. The study found that the immune response to Lyme disease is strongly age-related. Production of the cytokine IL-22 deceases with age, reducing the immune system's defenses against the *Borrelia* bacteria and creating a peak in the graph of infection rates. Researchers also found a genetic variation that increases production of the HIF-1a protein. This protein causes the amount of lactic acid in the cell to increase, which results in an energy deficiency in the immune cells. This triggers a reduction in

the production of IL-22 and other inflammatory proteins. *Borrelia* infections do not provide immunity from future infections. People with *Borrelia* antibodies in their blood did not have a stronger immune response to the bacteria than those that were sero-negative (Oosting, et al 2016).

In addition to Lyme disease, influenza epidemics and pandemics have been experienced since ancient times. The earliest historical description of an influenza outbreak may come from 412 BC. In an influenza pandemic, fifty percent or more of the population can be infected in a single year. An outbreak in 1580 represents the first well recorded flu epidemic. A strain emerged that summer in Asia, spread by land routes to Asia Minor and North Africa, before moving across Europe and into the Americas. Deaths were widely reported. The word "influenza" began to be used at that time. Since then, there have probably been fourteen or more influenza pandemics. In 1918, the worst influenza pandemic in recorded history killed an estimated fifty million people worldwide (Saunders-Hastings & Krewski, 2016).

Influenza pandemics,[from the Latin word *influentia* meaning "influence,"] are caused by a Type A strain of the virus. Type A is the only strain that also has an animal reservoir. Birds and swine get the flu. The highly variable nature of influenza genetic material prevents the maintenance of an adequate human immune response acquired through infections, leading to annual epidemics of various "seasonal influenza" and an annually changing modern vaccine. Like Lyme disease, exposure to flu does not lead to immunity to all flu.

The various epidemics that have occurred in the historic timespan, including the modern Lyme disease epidemic, can be theorized to have occurred in prehistory also. There is a natural survival process, with pathogens serving as a screening process. We are all mostly the children of survivors. Our genetic and epigenetic responses are generated by interactions with various bacteria, influenza, smallpox and various other viruses, and probably with others that are still unidentified. Some of these events are in the historical record, others have only been found by genetic research and by gaining knowledge of the immune system.

Any understanding of the human immune system requires a short trip back in time and a visit with some of our ancestors: Early Modern Humans, Neanderthals, and Denisovans, as well as other as yet unfound and unnamed Archaic Humans. Hominids may have developed in both Europe, as early as 9.7 years ago (Natural History Museum of Mainz, October 19, 2017) and in Africa (Johanson & Wong, 2010). Wherever they developed, humans have moved around alot. Hominids reached China by about 1.7 million years ago and Iberia by 1.4 million years ago.

Some Early Modern Humans that had evolved in Africa migrated by walking, either through the the Middle East or over a land bridge across a depleted Mediterranean Sea to Eurasia. When they arrived about 100,000 or so years ago, they mated with the Archaic Humans who were already there. Most modern humans outside Sub-Saharan Africa, as well as some groups in Africa, carry between one and four percent of inherited Neanderthal genetic material within their genome.

The amount of Archaic genes a person inherits depends upon where in the world they come from and whether their ancestors participated in several distinct episodes of interbreeding. Archeological evidence has found that Neanderthals had spread throughout Eurasia long before 200,000 years ago. Never a large group, there were probably never more than 70,000 Neanderthals alive at any point in time (O'Neill, 2011).The species became extinct by about 25,000 years ago, but not before they had shared some of their genes with ancient humans.

Neanderthal DNA survives today, most notably expressed in the skin, hair, and the immune systems of many humans. Neanderthal gene sequences are typically inherited in large batches, since they were injected into the modern human genome relatively recently and have not had time to break apart (Yong, E., 2014). Beginning at about 100,000 years ago (Kuhlwilm, 2016), Early Modern Humans acquired adaptive variants in some genes that must have conferred an advantage in their new locales because they have survived into modern times.

Today, the Neanderthal version of the skin gene POU2F3 is found in around sixty six percent of East Asians, while the

Neanderthal version of the gene BNC2, which affects skin color, is found in seventy percent of Europeans. But perhaps the most important genetic contributions were the Human Leukocyte Antigen [HLA] gene variants, which may explain why some people are better at fighting off some infections than others, but also contributes to increased susceptibility to autoimmune disease (Callaway, 2011). This is applicable to the modern Lyme disease epidemic. A Neanderthal version of Toll Like Receptors [TLR]1,6,10 that works in coordination with TLR2 may react more to Borrelia than a Human version because it has thousands of years more experience. Shared genes may indicate a process called cultural fusion(Danneman, et al, 2016).

There are various academic theories that have attempted to explain the development of human society. Perhaps the oldest is the Multi-Regional Hypothesis that claims that as different in appearance as modern humans, Neanderthals, Denisovans, and others might seem, they were all members of the same developing human species. Over eons, some traits predominated, but other traits that arose in localized environments and had adaptive value for that particular population were retained and bear some connection to human populations around the world today.

A starkly opposing theory has been driven by studies of the mitochondrial DNA of living populations. (Mitochondria are the organelles in cells that create chemical energy, carry their own unique sets of genes, and are passed on intact directly from mother to child). Those analyses suggest that the maternal bloodlines of every human alive today can be traced back to Africa at a time less than 100,000 years ago. This is the Out of Africa Model in which anatomically modern humans colonized Asia and Europe and displaced the Neanderthals and other Archaic Humans. The moderns may have directly exterminated the Archaics by introducing pathogens, through violence, or may simply have outcompeted with them for resources.

When, however, the painstaking work of recovering nuclear DNA from Neanderthal and Denisovan bones and sequencing it was done, it was determined that although we have no mitochondrial links or Y-haplotypes from the Archaics, on average

a proportion of many living human's genes, especially those with European or Asian ancestors, come from Archaic humans. This has led to a Fusion Theory, subscribed to by this author, that combines Multi-Regionalism with Out-of-Africanism. The Fusion Model begins with some hominids either developing in Europe or leaving Africa over 400,000 years ago and evolving over time into the Neanderthals and Denisovans who inhabited Europe and Central Asia. The hominids in Africa also evolved, mostly in the savannas of East Africa, into Early Modern Humans.

When some of these anatomically modern humans left Africa about 100,000 years ago, they mixed to a degree with the Archaic human populations but retained their own identity. Both the modern and archaic groups possessed locally varying patchworks of genetic traits and technologies that suited their distinct micro-environments creating the vibrant quilt of human culture that is constantly being constructed and re-constructed over time. Eventually, the Archaic human groups were fully assimilated by the Early Moderns with some of their genes persisting but disappeared as a separate distinct group. Neanderthals were extinct by 25,000 BP.

One of the most significant inheritances we received from our Archaic ancestors is our immune systems. When the *Borrelia* spiral, itself an ancient bacterial form, is injected into a modern human's body through tick attachment, it encounters an ancient set of defensive maneuvers that are the result of our species' experiences with pathogens over millennia. Called The Innate Immune System, it has a memory of the diseases that our ancestors encountered during their own lifetimes-even if the illness occurred thousands of years ago. Some of those memories come from Neanderthals. The Acquired or Adaptive Immune System, develops over a human lifetime in response to the various pathogens that a person encounters during individual experiences. The various cells of the immune system recognize and respond to pathogens in a generic way, by:

-recruiting immune cells to the site of infection by generating chemical signals called cytokines,

-by activating the complement cascade to identify bacteria, activate

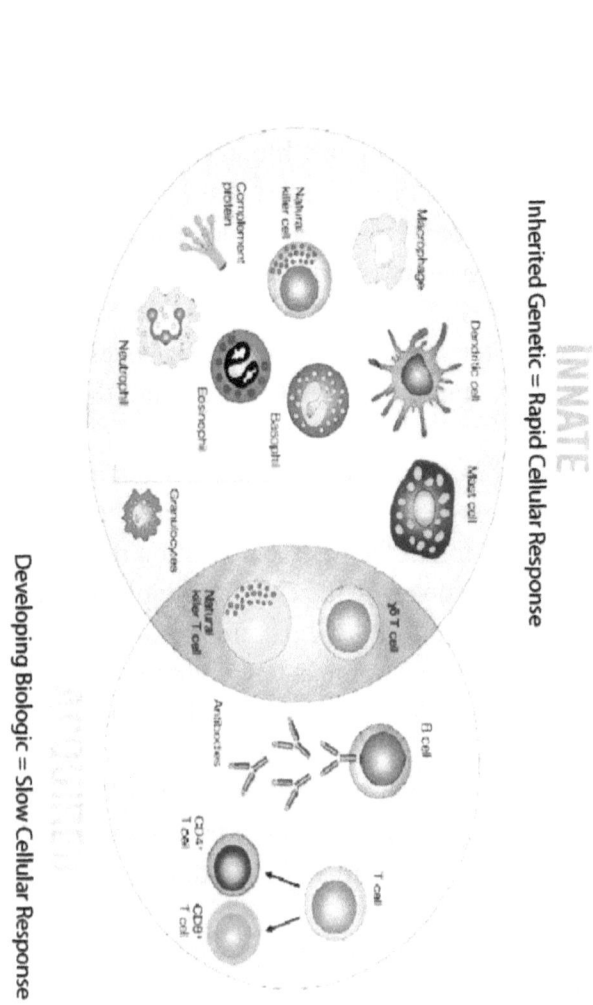

Figure 18. Cells involved in the Immune System. www.greensplus.com.

defense cells, and clear away dead cells and debris,
-acting as a chemical and physical barrier to infectious agents,
-alerting white blood cells to identify and remove foreign substances present in blood, organs, tissues and lymph system.

Neutrophils, specialized white blood cells, activate the Adaptive Immune System through a process known as antigen presentation. They surround potential pathogens and chemically break down their proteins into amino acid patterns, and then load the patterns onto Human Leukocyte Antigens (HLA) that display them to various Cluster of Determination (CD) genes which generate helper and suppressor T cells to confront the attacking pathogens.

Recognition of *Borrelia* by the immune system is mediated by pattern recognition receptors called Toll Like Receptors [TLR]. TLR2 has been found to be the main recognition receptor for *Borrelia*, but works in concert with TLR1, both playing a dominant role in the early response to *Borrelia* spirochetes. (Oosting, et al 2011). It turns out that some humans have inherited the Archaic variants of the set of Toll Like Receptor[TLR]group 1, 6, and 10, which cluster on the human fourth chromosome. These three TLRs are pre-programmed to trigger a rapid response to *Borrelia*, suggesting that the Neanderthals suffered from Lyme disease. But *Borrelia* also seem to know them and have developed a full bag of tricks to evade them.

Researchers suspect that for many years Neanderthal and Denisovan populations in Europe and Asia confronted various pathogens and were selectively winnowed down to only those individuals best able to cope with the environment and unique constellation of pathogens in their regions. The lower seasonal levels of sunlight available in northern latitudes shaped genetic variations among Neanderthals-especially in skin pigmentation. Having lived in Eurasia for thousands of years before the arrival of the first humans from Africa, Neanderthals were adapted to low sunlight levels and Vitamin D processing with lighter skin. These adaptions were passed on to Early Modern Humans. Sun exposure may have shaped Neanderthal phenotypes and that gene flow continues to contribute to variation in these human traits today.

Skin and hair color, circadian rhythms, and mood are all influenced by sunlight exposure.

When Early Modern Humans moved into an area and mingled with the Archaic inhabitants, they produced children who inherited immunity genes that were better attuned to the local environment and were more likely to survive. In this way the modern human genome received and retained an unusually large dose of Archaic genes that improved immunity (Dannemann, M. & Kelso, J., October 5, 2017).The modern Innate Immune System is a fusion of human and Archaic human genes.

The Innate Immune System is designed to mount a fast response to potentially dangerous invaders. A newborn would otherwise have little defense against life-threatening infections. People of any age, encountering infectious agents that their bodies have never met before, would be in big trouble if it were not for this first line of defense. Present at birth, Toll Like Receptors are already programmed to recognize basic patterns of microbial presence. Some TLRs sit astride cell membranes and others reside inside cells, each alert to the presence of viruses, bacteria, fungi, and other microbial invaders that slip past the skin and mucous membranes. Once they detect an invader, TLRs can trigger a number of responses to destroy the microbial interloper.

The Adaptive Immune System is trained as a human matures. Part of that training comes from actual exposure to microbes and other irritants. While TLR's are the first-responders, they also help educate the cells of the Adaptive Immune System. To do this, TLRs prompt dendritic cells to capture some of the invading material and to present it to the cells of the Adaptive Immune System, which develops antibodies to common infections after the first exposure. The Adaptive Immune System requires time to do this. Ultimately, though, it provides our bodies with a long-lasting, targeted defense against specific pathogens.

Archaic versions of TLR1,6, and10 can sometimes go awry and cause allergies by over-reacting to non-threatening entities, like pollen. But they are also protective. In one study, people with these archaic TLR clusters have lower levels of the bacterium *Helicobacter pylori* (M. Deschamps et al., 2016).

Human genetic history is complex. In northern climates, the story is punctuated by periods of glaciation related isolation. The complete Neanderthal genome was sequenced in 2013 by extracting DNA from a 50,000 year old bone that archeologists had uncovered in Siberia. By comparing the modern human genome to the Neanderthals, they found that eight percent of the Neanderthal DNA comes from yet another unknown group of Archaic Humans, a hint that other unknown groups in Asia and Africa also left genes in modern humans.

By April of 2014, a first glimpse into the epigenetics and a map of the full methylation process for Neanderthal and Denisovan DNA had been produced. This map allowed researchers to assess Archaic gene activity levels and compare them to modern humans. Again, the most significant findings were related to disease and the immune systems. Researchers reported that Neanderthal DNA sequences still strongly influence how our genes are turned on or off. Neanderthal effects on gene expression also contribute to physical traits like height as well as susceptibility to schizophrenia, lupus, osteoporosis, blood-coagulation disorders, biliary cirrhosis, Crohn's disease, type 2 diabetes and even nicotine addiction (Cell, 2016). Researchers have shown that nine previously identified human genetic variants that are associated with specific traits came from Neanderthals. All humans differ in the outcome that follows exposure to pathogens because of this complex ancestry. Most Africans, however, do not have any Archaic genes. This effects immune reactions.

One recent study, using RNA sequencing, looked at the response of primary monocytes from Africans and Europeans when confronted by bacterial and viral stimuli. Toll-like receptor pathways (TLR1/2, TLR4, and TLR7/8) were stimulated using influenza virus. Marked differences in immune responses were detected within and between populations, with a strong hot spot at TLR 1 that decreased the expression of pro-inflammatory genes in Europeans only. This difference may or may not be linked with a particular viral outbreak that occurred in Europe at some point in past time.

Researchers found that one Neanderthal gene called OAS1-3

was twenty seven times more active than the European human version within two hours of infection with influenza or herpes simplex 1 and 2, quickly halting infection. Another study found that PNMA1, a gene that produces a protein that directly interacts with the flu virus, is super enriched in the Neanderthal genes that are present in thirty three percent of all Europeans. This may be the result of survival from the deadly influenza epidemics of the past (Houldcroft & Underdown, 2016).

    For some diseases, a programmed immune response tends to help with survival, for others it can be detrimental. Regulatory variants in European genomes slow some responses. On the other hand, genetically driven immune systems that produce higher rates of inflammation may explain why African American women are up to three times more prone to the autoimmune disease Lupus (Reardon, 2016, Riley, 2017). Humans have a history of moving around. People have migrated around so much in the last four or five centuries that the human immune system has not always kept pace with change. There sometimes appears to be a mismatch between environment and immune system that only time can heal.

    For example, modern Sub-Saharan Africans carry a mutation to a gene known as DARC, which provides resistance to malaria [*Plasmodium vivax*], which is common in Africa. Malaria normally uses DARC to enter red blood cells. In the past, people carrying the DARC mutation were better able to survive, reproduce, and passed along the mutation to their descendants. Unfortunately, the DARC mutation carries a side effect that has been devastating in modern times. It makes people more susceptible to HIV infection. Men with the DARC mutation are forty percent more likely to have acquired HIV. This genetic vulnerability may account for about eleven percent of all HIV infection on the African continent (Ledford, 2008).

    On the other hand, a genetic mutation in a chemokine receptor called CCR5 delta 32 provides people who carry two copies of it with almost complete protection from human immunodeficiency virus [HIV]. It also seems to hamper the development of several other pathogens. The mutation mediates the entry of poxviruses into target cells and slows the progression of multiple sclerosis. One consequence of any CCR5 deficiency is a more robust T-cell response and the generation of more dendritic cells in the lymph nodes. This creates an enhanced response to mycobacterium tuberculosis, listeria, and lymphocytic *choriomeningitis* viral infections. This T-cell response also facilitates recovery from hepatitis B (Thio, 2007).

    The mutation seems to have appeared in Northern Europe about 5000 years ago and probably offered some benefit against pox infections. It has risen to relatively high frequency and is carried by five to fourteen percent of the modern European population. But although providing protection against HIV, it has a deleterious role in other pathologies. Patients have been found to be at higher risk for symptomatic West Nile Virus and tick-borne encephalitis TBEV[both *flaviviruses*](Kindberg, 2008). The lack of CCR5 may serve as an unlocked door for cell invasion by *flaviviruses*. In this case, the immune system seems experienced at handling retroviruses like HIV but less adept at handing *flaviviruses*. Traces of past experience still haunt the present!

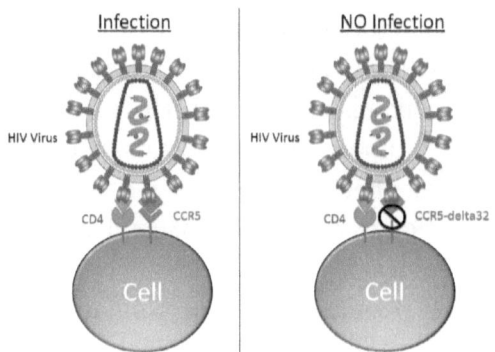

Figure 19. How HIV infects cells, using CD4 and CCR5 receptors. www.theodysseyonline.com.

    European and African populations also have statistically different responses to Lyme disease-fewer African Americans contract it but when they do it is severe. This has been explained in the United States as being part of a suburban/urban environmental risk divide. African Americans who contract Lyme disease were, in one study, ten percent more likely to develop

neurological and heart problems and thirty percent more likely to suffer from Lyme induced arthritis. A significant difference was also found in the rate of the Bulls Eye Rash[EM], which is blamed on darker skin colorings obscuring the rash. Among all patients, there was a significant negative association between the notation of rash [which may have triggered earlier treatment] and arthritis. Although much of the racial disparity in incidence rates diminishes in a rural endemic area, a difference still remains. This may be attributed to a hyperactive Innate Immune System's causing reactive damage (Fix, et al, 2000).

African-American males are also at particular risk for serious complications from *Rickettsia* [Rocky Mountain spotted fever], as they are genetically more likely to be deficient in glucose-6-phosphate dehydrogenase (G6PD), an enzyme associated with the maintenance of membrane integrity in red blood cells (Chen & Sexton, 2008).

There are many other factors that influence the progression of Lyme disease. One of the most important is the Human Leukocyte Antigen complex. HLA helps the immune system distinguish the body's own proteins from the proteins of foreign invaders. Within one class of HLA genes, researchers estimate that Europeans owe half of their variants to interbreeding with Archaic humans, Asians owe up to eighty percent, and Papua New Guineans up to ninety five percent. Increasingly, autoimmune diseases have been recognized as having a genetic basis that is mediated by HLA subtypes.

Archaic HLA genes create a genetic disposition towards development of autoimmune disease, typically requiring some environmental trigger to evolve into a full-blown disease. For instance, celiac disease has been strongly associated with HLA-DQ2, and Type I diabetes, rheumatoid arthritis, Lyme arthritis and multiple sclerosis with HLA-DR4. In mouse studies, HLA-DR4 has been found to be an indicator of Chronic Lyme Disease. When infected with *Borrelia*, mice with HLA-DR 4 produced an inflammatory immune response that generated lots of interferon gamma but no antibodies to the spirochetes.(Iliopoulou, Alroy & Huber, 2008).

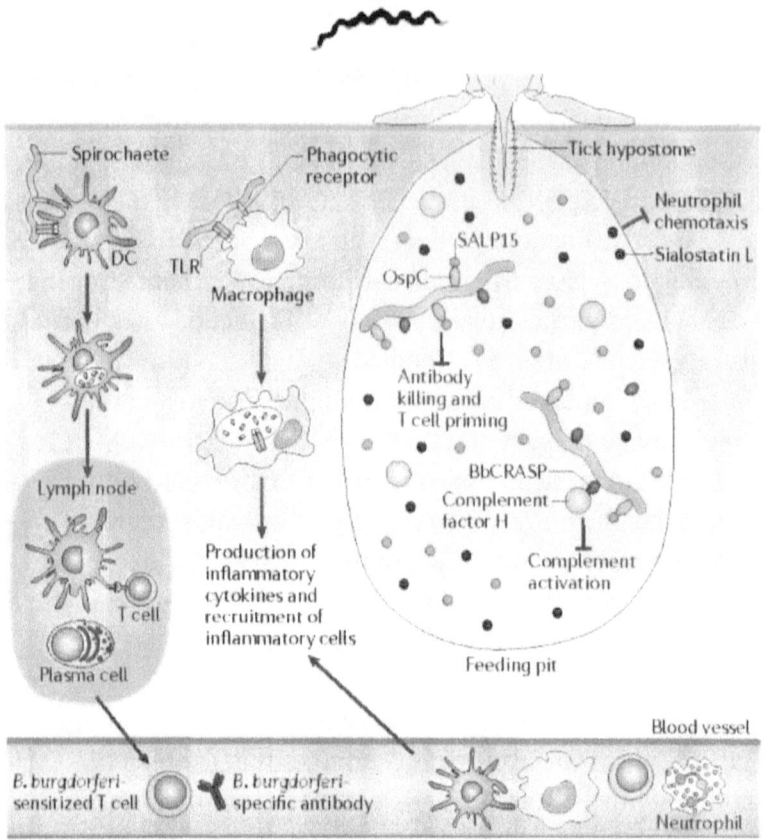

Figure 20. The tick-mammal interface. Borrelia have been evading mammal immune systems for thousands of years. A tick creates a feeding pit with its barbed hypostome mouth and anchors to the skin of a blood meal host. Initial salivary secretions form a cement cone around the attachment site that further anchors the tick. The tick injects a blob of saliva containing a plethora of bioactive agents which *Borrelia burgdorferi* exploits to help establish infection. These include OSP binding to SALP15, masking the spirochetes from attacking antibodies, as well as sialostatin L, which blocks neutrophil chemotaxis. A group of *borrelial* surface lipoproteins called BbCRASP bind to complement Factor H, which delays activation of the complement pathway. When *Borrelia* cells are finally recognized via pattern recognition receptors, they are taken within phagolysomes to the lymph nodes where processed *borrelial* antigens are displayed to T and B cells which alert system effector cells to the pathogens. Immune system cells which are sensitized by T cells, accompanied by pro-inflammatory cytokines, recruited neutrophils, and macrophages migrate to the site of the tick attachment. This can lead to an Erythema Migrans [Bull's-Eye] rash. The TLR forms that humans inherited from the Neanderthals recognize *Borrelia*. From Rudolf, et al., 2012.

When challenged by the human immune system, *Borrelia* have a few survival tricks up their metaphorical spiral sleeves that they have learned over millenia. During their transfer from tick[*Ixodes scapularis or Ixodes ricinus]* to human, *Borrelia* bind to a substance called Salivary Protein 15[Salp15] that is excreted in the midgut of the tick. This masks their Outer Surface Proteins [OSP], making the newly arrived bacteria virtually invisible to the Innate Immune System and protecting them from complement system attack (Schuijt, 2008). Immune antibody responses are delayed until the Salp15 degrades and the bacteria's own OSP become detectable. This gives *Borrelia* an infective head start as it makes its way into human tissues.

When the invading bacteria is finally detected, the Innate Immune System launches a strong cascade of proteins from the complement system. This system unleashes attack complexes that can dismantle invading microbes. It does not damage the body's own cells because they are tagged with an identifying marker called Factor H. *Borrelia* have mastered the ability to get inside a cell and bind to Factor H, which again allows them to evade the immune system. OSP can also bind to plasminogen, which activates an enzyme known as plasmin, which the spirochetes use to break down barriers to deep tissue invasion.

Plasmin activates other enzymes known as collagenases and matrix metallproteinases. These help the Borrelia penetrate the otherwise impenetrable tight junctions that protect tissues from unwanted guests. *Borrelia* cause structural abnormalities in "germinal centers,"sites in the lymph nodes and lymph tissues that are key to producing a long term protective immune response. Infection seems to prevent these germinal centers from producing B cells and antibodies that are crucial for the immune systems's memory formation creating immunity against future infections. Researchers found that a *Borrelia burgdorferi* infection even prevented induction of a strong response to an influenza infection (Bailey, 2015). In this way, Lyme disease may increase the severity of other infections.

Borrelia have an ability to switch out a variety of Outer Surface Proteins. It can bleb off tiny bits of OSP to confuse

immune cells and also produces different presenting VlsE antigens. When many VlsE antigens are processed and presented to T helper cells, the information is translated into antibody-producing B cells that produce the IgG antibodies that patrol the body for any signs of that particular VlsE antigen target. When variation in VlsE antigens occurs, the result is a weak, poorly focused antibody response. Confused B cells end up with nothing to do but pile up within the lymph nodes.

    Genes play a role in this myriad of components involved in this human immune system. Cytokines are proteins that serve as molecular messengers between cells. Cytokines regulate inflammatory responses. They regulate the body's response to disease and infection, as well as mediate normal cellular processes in the body. There are both pro-inflammatory cytokines and anti-inflammatory cytokines. The pro-inflammatory cytokines play a role in the development of inflammatory and neuropathic pain. The anti-inflammatory cytokines are immune antagonists. Overproduction or inappropriate production of certain cytokines by the body can result in disease. There is evidence to suggest that they are involved in initiating pain as well as in the persistence of pain. Scientists have found that seventeen immune-system signaling proteins in the blood correlate with the severity of chronic fatigue. This reflects different genetic predispositions among patients (McInnes I. and Schett G.. 2007 and Zhang, 2007).

    Located on Chromosome 1, an inherited genetic code that may effect the course of Lyme disease for some people is MTHFR- the genes which encode and direct methylenetetrahydrofolate reductase production [an enzyme]. These genes are directly responsible for producing glutathione-the body's master detoxification agent. MTHFR adds a methyl group to folate [vitamin B9]with the help of vitamin B6 and B12, to make it usable by the body. It is important for converting the amino acid cysteine into methionine, which the body needs for proper metabolism and muscle growth. MTHFR directs a metabolic process that repairs DNA, switches genes on and off, and has numerous other important functions (Nazki, F.H. Et al, 2014). People with MTHFR polymorphisms may have trouble effectively

eliminating toxins. This may also contribute to the prevalence of Chronic Lyme symptoms.

The MTHFR mutations that have the greatest influence on human health are: homozygous C677T and compound heterozygous with A1298C. It is thought that these mutations can inhibit MTHFR enzyme function by up to a whopping seventy percent (Bezold, G. et al, 2001). Once again, MTHFR genes and polymorphisms have been linked to our Archaic ancestors. While MTHFR C677T seems to have spread out of Africa, the A1298C genetic variant has been found in Neanderthal genomes (Lowry et al., 2013).These mutations create an elevated level of the enzyme homocysteine in the blood, increasing risk for several medical conditions: cardiovascular disorders, atherosclerosis, myocardial infarction, stroke, minimal cognitive impairment, dementia, Parkinson's disease, multiple sclerosis, epilepsy, and eclampsia. There is evidence from laboratory and clinical studies that the condition exerts direct toxic effects on both the vascular and nervous systems (Ansari,et al., 2014).

The distributions of these two MTHFR variants are quite high and may be involved in Lyme disease presentation. Overall, about eighty five percent of the general population carries at least one of these variants. They may or may not be protective against *Borrelia*. The genotype frequencies for MTHFR are high among East Asians, with a frequency exhibited that increases in the southern-central-northern direction in Mainland China, which mirrors tick-borne infection rates.The frequency of the MTHFR A1298C polymorphism exhibits the reverse trend, decreasing from southern to central to northern China. In Europe, a north-to-south increase in the frequency of the 677T allele has also been observed. The methylation process in disease response is still poorly understood, but it has been found that some ancient DNA has been directing this epigenetic mechanism since lives were lived thousands of years ago (Briggs, et al., 2009).

Tracing those lives and the lives of the cluster of other species created modern humans is key to understanding both the past and the present. Migratory activity is a critical factor in shaping processes of both biological and cultural change through

time. Human Immune Responses vary depending not only upon the present lived experiences of the individual but also upon the pathogens encountered by their ancestors. This may be another reason why "one size fits all treatment regiments" for Lyme disease have such a high failure rate.

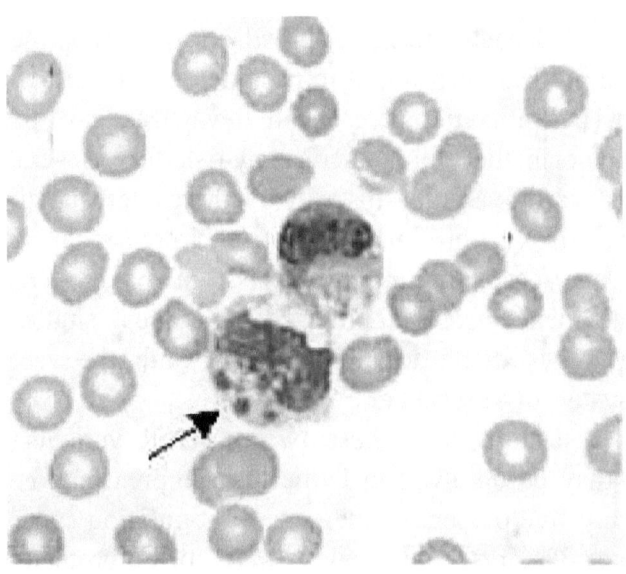

Figure 21. Anaplasma multiplies into a granulocyte after burrowing within the immune system's white blood cells called neutrophils. www. infection landscapes.org.

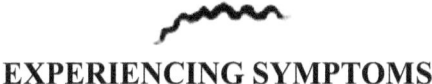
EXPERIENCING SYMPTOMS

Lyme disease is an extremely frustrating ailment to describe because it presents with such a diverse variety of symptoms. Because so many body systems can become involved, Lyme disease can take on a wide array of forms. In a very small number of people, it is an extremely severe pathology and can be fatal, especially if the heart muscle is infected or pneumonia develops. However, it is believed that prior to the establishment of an antibiotic protocol for Lyme disease it was generally a mild and occasionally a miserable but, in normal circumstances, survivable condition.

In one sad study, ninety patients in the former Soviet Union with Bull's Eye rashes and flu-like symptoms that developed after documented tick bites were studied, *but not treated with antibiotics*. This study provides a good outline of symptoms that the infected would have displayed in the past. Within two weeks to four months of infection, sixty-four percent of the patients had developed neurological abnormalities, including cranial neuritis, Bell's palsy, meningitis, or radicular pain. Four percent developed arthritis. In another study of patients with Lyme meningitis, it was found that, without antibiotics, the duration of neurological involvement was three to eighteen months. Untreated Lyme disease may have been responsible for many of the rheumatic conditions, aches, pains, dementia and mental illness that were sometimes thought to be a normal part of the aging process in the past in endemic areas (Anan'eva et al.,1995).

This diversity of symptoms may be in and of itself diagnostic of the affliction. Dr. Brian Fallon, the director of the Lyme and Tick-borne Diseases Research Center at Columbia University Medical Center, has suggested that if symptoms involving more than one specific bodily system are present, Lyme disease should at the very least be considered. "There are not many things that can cause brain problems and joint problems at the same time," he said (Fallon, et al. 1992).

Some hormonal responses, however, especially those associated with menstruation, stress, or a weakened host immune

system, seem to trigger an "all clear to revert to spirochete again" signal. So can the arrival of a new set of bacteria from a subsequent tick bite. One recent study found that *Borrelia* spirochetes participate in a form of mating that transfers genetic material in the process. Previously cyst encased *Borrelia* within a host's body may sense the Outer Surface Proteins of newly arrived bacteria and transform into spirochetes to meet, mix and mingle with the newly arrived .

The experience of Lyme disease can be understood by looking at the medical and scientific literature but it is also a very idiosyncratic condition that can be best described by the person experiencing the symptom or by an observer of the afflicted. A growing body of modern source material can be found that includes descriptions of the experiences of Lyme disease.

Lyme disease can be accompanied by seizures. The mother of a teenager from an endemic area of New Jersey described the seizures that he developed after contracting Lyme disease. He had "episodes of tremors, wherein his body would shake and twitch uncontrollably"(Lang, 2004).

Most modern Lyme patients live lives of relative obscurity. But in some famous cases, the disease has played out across the pages of national newspapers. Former President George W. Bush has been infected, as have Senator Chuck Shumer of New York and former Governor Christy Whitman of New Jersey. Darryl Hall, of the singing group Hall and Oates, was forced to cancel a concert tour after contracting the disease writing "I used to think I had allergies, because I used to feel feverish," he said. "And then one day I got a really high fever, my neck stiffened up, I had all kinds of aches and pains and I got really bad tremors"(www.huffingtonpost.com, July 22, 2016). The promising career of golfer Tim Herron was sidelined by severe fatigue and what felt like a sinus infection, cold sweats, and a full body rash in 2004. It took a string of emergency room visits and four doctor's opinions before he was diagnosed with Lyme disease (http://www.asapsports.com, 2004, August 29).

In June of 2005, Wyatt Sexton, a quarterback for the Florida State University football team, was found disheveled and

disoriented lying on a street in Tallahassee. He identified himself as God and was taken to a hospital after being doused with pepper spray by the local police. At first, some form of drug abuse was suspected because these aberrant symptoms had appeared so rapidly. Eventually, he was found to have an active Lyme disease infection that had resulted in neuro-psychiatric and cardiovascular deficits(http://www.sun-sentinel.com, 2005, June 6). Phil Bredesen, while Governor of Tennessee, contracted a "sudden acute illness" that may have been tick-bite related (http://www.foxnews.com/2006, August 16).

Polly Murray contracted Lyme disease over thirty years ago. She lived in Lyme, Connecticut where she, her husband, and three of her children may have been infected by the disease sometime before the early 1970's. Her work, along with many others, in trying to find answers to what was happening within her family and community, has been key to raising scientific and public awareness of this disease. Her book, *The Widening Circle,* is an autobiographical account of her own experiences with Lyme disease.

Another well-documented modern experience with Lyme disease comes from the novelist Amy Tan, who was diagnosed with a case that had advanced into late stage symptoms. She has been very vocal about its devastating effects. She suffered from hallucinations (usually at night when she was in bed) which she has described. Once she saw a naked man approaching her bed and thought it was her husband. "It was the middle of the night," and "he wasn't saying anything or doing anything else. He was just coming toward me (before stopping) next to the bed stand, as though he was turning on the light." She "thought someone was dead. I reached for him and the image started to warp as I realized he wasn't real." The experience was terrifying. Amy Tan's other symptoms have included hair loss, fatigue, tinnitus, memory loss, olfactory hallucinations, and the misspelling of words when writing. When speaking, even after antibiotic treatment, she sometimes replaces words with similar sounding gibberish (McCoy, 2003).

Actor Alec Baldwin suffered from Lyme disease symptoms every August for five years, "The first time was the worst of all," Baldwin said, describing "black lung, flu-like symptoms, sweating to death in my bed." He remembered thinking at the time, "I'm not going to live," and "I'm going to die of Lyme disease"(Young, 2017).

Ms. Nicole Greene serves as an Office of Women's Health spokesperson for the United States government. She writes: "On Easter Sunday 2007, I woke up unable to move from the neck down. My doctor tested me for all sorts of things: lupus, fibromyalgia, chronic fatigue syndrome, multiple sclerosis, sickle cell disease. But only one test came back positive: Lyme disease. After my diagnosis, I thought through my entire medical history. I realized that I had actually had a lot of symptoms — I just didn't know they were symptoms. I was sick all the time. None of my doctors ever put all of my symptoms together. But once I was diagnosed with Lyme disease, it all made much more sense.I immediately went on antibiotics, which wiped me out so much that I couldn't go into the office, or even the grocery store. I was lucky to be able to work from home, but many people don't have that option. For almost a year, I missed a lot of things — my friends, family, birthday parties, celebrations, saying goodbye to loved ones who passed away. That first year was really hard.Even after I started feeling better, my body wasn't completely well… I've dealt with sciatica, a spinal lesion, neuropathy, temporary hair loss, cognitive issues, stress fractures in both knees … Lyme has affected my body, my work, and my relationships…. I've learned about chronic Lyme disease, its co-infections, and new options for treatment… A lot of Lyme-literate doctors don't take insurance, and all of the appointments, blood work, and treatments are out of pocket and very expensive. …my family and I have made sacrifices to ensure that I have the resources to make those choices… It's been 15 years now, but I'm finally living with my Lyme disease." (https://www.womenshealth.gov/blog/my-life-lyme).

Singer Avril Lavigne was diagnosed with Lyme disease in 2014 after suffering from bouts of extreme exhaustion.I n an

interview with People Magazine, Lavigne said that she'd been lethargic and bedridden for five months. "I couldn't breathe, I couldn't talk and I couldn't move," she said in the interview. "I thought I was dying."In a later interview with *Good Morning America*, Lavigne spoke more about her battle with the disease. "I'd wake up and have night sweats and I felt like I had the flu," she said. "This went on and off for a month." After seeing numerous specialists who misdiagnosed her, the singer ultimately found a Lyme disease specialist and is expected to make a full recovery (Marcus, 2015).

"I have lost the ability to read, write, or even watch TV, because I can't process information or any stimulation for that matter," Yolanda Foster of *The Real Housewives of Beverly Hills* fame said in the post. "It feels like someone came in and confiscated my brain and tied my hands behind my back just to see life go by without me participating in it.The most frustrating part of this disease is that you look so normal from the outside" (Rice, 2015).

The former *The Sopranos* and *Entourage* star Jamie Lynn Sigler contracted Lyme disease while filming a movie in rural New Jersey. Luckily, Sigler is an example of successful treatment after early detection: the actress first noticed a tingling sensation in her feet and shortly after, she experienced paralysis of her legs. After spending five days in a hospital, doctors diagnosed her with Lyme disease and she was given antibiotic treatment, which was effective in combating the disease."It was such a life-altering experience," Sigler said in a 2001 interview with the *Newark Star Ledger.* "I realized it could all be taken away in a moment. It's hard to explain, when you sit there and can't move anything."

Bella Hadid spoke to the British magazine *Evening Standard* about her 2012 diagnosis. "I stopped driving because I kept crashing, because my brain just stopped working," she said. "I was exhausted all the time. It affected my memory so I suddenly wouldn't remember how to drive to Santa Monica from Malibu where I lived"(Hadid, 2017).

Kelly Osbourne would write "What annoys me is that this is a real, real disease," she explained. "It almost killed me. I will do

anything to raise awareness for it, because I almost died from it, and it's a debilitating disease that most of the time goes misdiagnosed." In 2004, Kelly she was bitten by a tick. Her dad burned it off with a match and that, she thought, was the end of that. But in the years that followed, she suffered from persistent body aches, headaches, stomach pain and trouble sleeping. In 2013, she had a seizure on the set of a show. As her symptoms piled up, so did the prescriptions: Ambien, Trazodone, anti-seizure medications, even painkillers, despite her past addiction issues. The pills robbed her of her energy and emotions. "You know in movies where a mental patient sits in a rocking chair in a cardigan and nightgown and stares at a wall all day?" Osbourne has written in her memoir, *There Is No F*cking Secret: Letters From a Badass Bitch,* "that was me!" She kept her diagnosis private, she writes, "not only for fear of pharmaceutical companies coming after me because of the cure I found in Germany but also because it seems like the trendy disease to have right now."

Since being diagnosed in 2013, Debbie Gibson has been fighting the bacterial infection but has appeared on Dancing With the Stars. Her dance partner writes:"It's one thing to heal from a disease like Lyme disease, where it's excruciating on your body, but another thing to do it on live television, so it's very inspirational that she's even trying to do this. She's inspiring me -- and hopefully Americans who are going to be watching- to get up and really try to get back to the good place in your life"(www.etonline.com, video 87176).

When Martha Stewart told David Letterman, who had just contracted Lyme disease, that she has had it "a dozen times," she was speaking for a significant group of Lyme patients who usually go un-noticed. Lyme can be a recurring nightmare and for every celebrity story told, there are thousands of past and present Lyme altered lives whose stories will never be told.

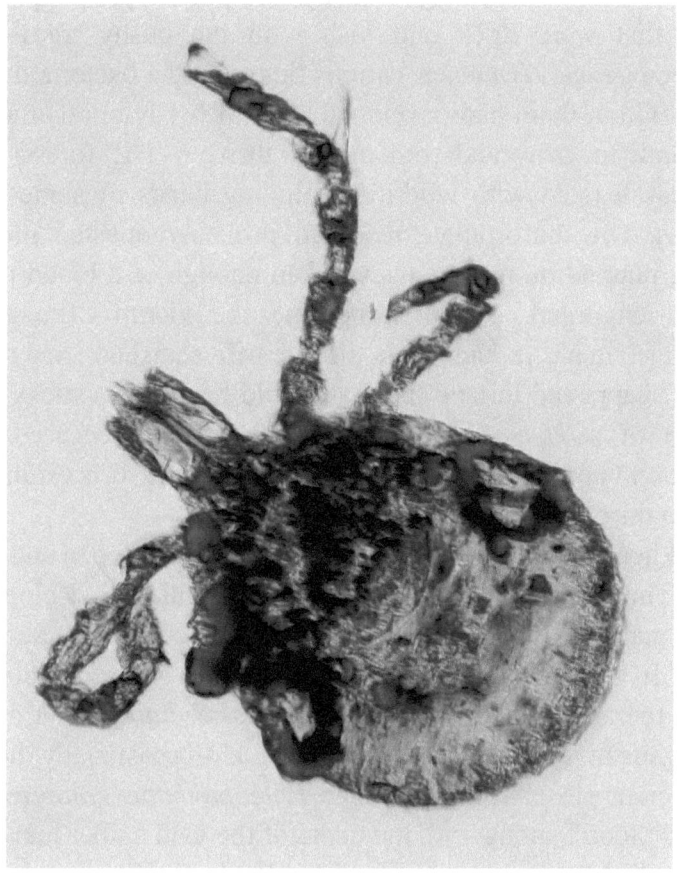

Figure 22. Ancient *Paleoborrelia* were found inside an ancient *Ixodes* tick fossilized in amber, like this one. Credit: George Poinar, Jr., Oregon State University, 2014.

QUESTING FOR DINOSAURS

Both the *Borrelia* spirochete and the *Ixodes* ticks that vector them are ancient, tried and true organism forms that developed long before humans evolved. Bacteria are probably the most ancient group of lifeforms on earth, dating back to about 3.6 billion years ago-almost as old as the planet itself. Ticks carry a number of bacterial pathogens and appear to have done so for millions of years. We know this because ticks have been found in a very ancient context-amber.

The amber story begins many millions of years ago within forests that were thick and lush with the bushy trees of the evergreen genus, *Hymenea*. Various ticks and the bacteria that they carried within them had developed a set of behaviors that allowed them both to grow and sometimes thrive. The forests of the Americas teamed with wildlife, including bands of some sort of primates. One unfortunate tick had probably quested in a low branch, jumped on to a monkey, taken enough of a blood meal to become engorged, and then became the victim of a primate grooming ritual. It had been picked off, squished, and thrown away. It happened to land in what would become its sticky grave- the sap of a *Hymenea* tree. The tick became encased as an inclusion in amber that was later found in a mine. It is estimated to be up to thirty million years old.

When it was thrown away, the tick had burst open and leaked blood. Those spots of blood are the first fossilized red blood cells from a mammal that have ever been discovered. They had a story to tell. It was one of a long ago infection. The red blood cells carried the ancestors of a modern piroplasm, *Babesia,* a malaria-like organism. It infects livestock, pets, and occasionally, humans. The ancient piroplasm was named *Paleohaimatus calabresi,* latin for "old blood" along with the name of the avid amber hunter who had supplied the specimen tacked on (Zhang, 2017).

Amber is found in deposits in many places. In Europe, especially in the Baltic area, the deposits are thought to be fossil resin remains of the now extinct *Sciadopityaceae* family of plants. By examining inclusions in amber, scientists have found that the relationship between bacteria and various insects and ticks has been going on in the earth's forests for millennia. They have, for example, found a flea with the remnants of an ancient form of *Yersinia*, the bacteria that causes the plague, stuck to its proboscis and rectum after a blood meal. While human strains of *Yersinia pestis* could well have evolved only in the past 10,000 to 20,000 years, ancient strains could have evolved as rodent parasites.

As soft-bodied forms, bacteria are rarely preserved in the record. Amber is the exception. Amber is a semi-precious stone that

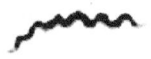

Babesia infect red blood cells, creating a maltese cross pattern. Ancient red blood cells found within a fossilized tick show similar infection.

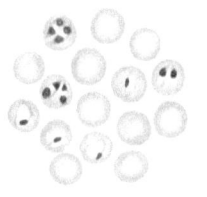 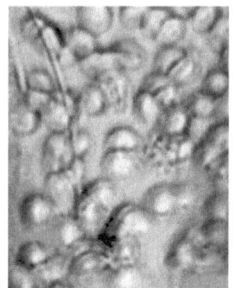

Figures 23. Fossilized blood cells infected with Babesia. Credit: George Poinar, Jr., Oregon State University, 2014.

begins as free-flowing tree sap and slowly turns into a hard mineral. An ancient spirochete with characteristics of *Borrelia* was found in a larval tick belonging to the genus *Iyomma* (Arachnida: Ixodidae) from a piece of amber that had been mined in the Dominican Republic. This shows that a *Borrelia*-like spiral shaped bacteria has been lurking inside the guts of ticks for more than fifteen million years. The size and shape of the fossil spirochetes closely resemble those of the present-day *Borrelia* species. This finding has helped scientists trace the evolution of pathogen–vector associations. They may have begun when the spirochetes came into contact with tick eggs that were deposited in soil or leaf litter. When *Borrelia* began as a tick parasite, it could have been passed from mother to offspring by vertical or transovarial transmission (TOT) as symbionts. A later evolutionary step involved entering the tick salivary glands where they could be transferred to vertebrates.

The presence of spirochetes in the hemocoel [a cavity in an open circulatory system that bathes the organs directly with oxygen and nutrients] of the fossilized tick shows that it was already a competent vector host millions of years ago. The vertebrate blood meal hosts of extant *Ixodes* ticks are reptiles, birds and mammals. Remains of all three groups, including feathers and rodent hairs, have also been found in Dominican amber. It is likely that the genetic matter from this spirochete contributed to the evolution of the modern *Borrelia* that infect humans. The ancient

spirochete have been labeled as fossil genus and species *Palaeoborrelia dominicanan* (Poinar, 2014).

Starting at this point in time, and adding the fact that the *Ixodes* tick developed a life cycle that includes a state of overwintering in temperate forest leaf litter, a molecular clock for the evolution of the housekeeping genes of the causative agent of Lyme disease in humans has not yet been fully established (Margos, et al, 2008). Nor has its place of origins been pinpointed. Various lineages of the pathogen separated a few millions of years ago. There is strong evidence of prehistoric population size expansion in North America and an east-to-west radiation of descendent clades from founding sequence types in the North East. *Borrelia burgdorferi* was present in North America many thousands of years before European settlements. *Borrelia* populations have been found to have recently reemerged independently out of separate relict foci (Hoena et al., 2009).

Other ancient pathogens has also been found with fossilized ticks. *Rickettsia-like* organisms within a one hundred million year old tick was found in fossilized amber that was mined in Myanmar, Southeast Asia. *Rickettsia* is an infection that causes modern diseases like Rocky Mountain Spotted Fever and Typhus. Various studies infer a Jurassic/Cretaceous split into *Rickettsia* bacteria associated with protozoans and a lineage more typical for blood sucking arthropods. Molecular studies report a rapid radiation of this bacterial genus among blood-feeding taxa going back to about 50–65 million years ago, contemporary with a radiation of possible mammalian blood meal hosts.

Rickettsia is named after the scientist Howard Taylor Ricketts (1871–1910), who studied spotted fever in the Bitterroot Valley of Montana. The *Rickettsiae* are a diverse group of bacteria, some of which can be transmitted to humans via the bites of ticks, fleas, lice or mites. Rocky Mountain spotted fever was originally called Black Measles because patients develop a characteristic spotted rash appearance throughout their body.

It may have occurred in the historical past but the first clinical description of *Rickettsia* was written in 1899. Ricketts characterized the basic epidemiological features of the disease

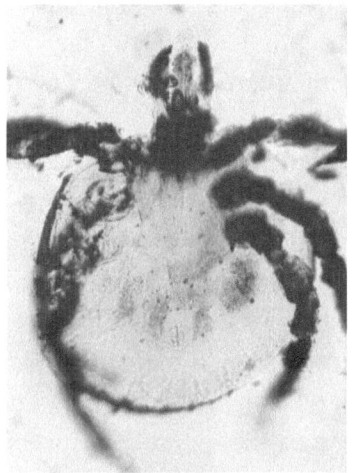 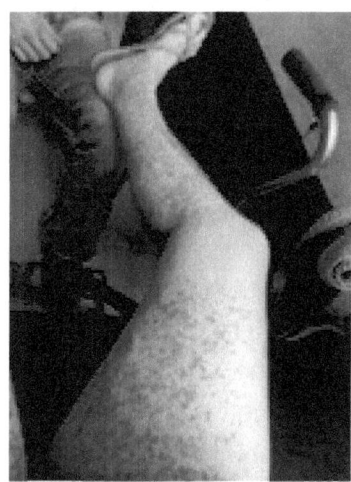

Figures 24. *Rickettsia*-like cells were found in the body cavity of a 100 million year old Myanmar amber larval tick, *Cornupalpatum burmanicum (Ixodida: Ixodidae)*. The size and shape of the fossil cells resemble those of present day members of the *Rickettsiaceae* bacteria family. Credit: George Poinar, Jr., Oregon State University, 2014. Rickettsia causes Rocky Mountain fever, which is accompanied by a severe rash. Facebook public posting 10/2017.

including the role of tick vectors. Untreated *Rickettsia* has an 80-90% mortality rate (Steele, 2005). The disease is mentioned in the 1866 book *Cradock Nowell: A Tale of the New Forest*. African-American males are at particular risk for serious complications of Rocky Mountain spotted fever, as they are genetically more likely to be deficient in glucose-6-phosphate dehydrogenase (G6PD), an enzyme associated with the maintenance of membrane integrity in red blood cells. Prior to the antibiotic era, Rocky Mountain spotted fever had a mortality rate of up to thirty percent. Even today, it remains the most common fatal tick-borne disease in the United States.

It may have 'bugged' the dinosaurs. By studying the mouth parts of ticks, it has been found that they evolved early and would have been able to pierce through even the thickest of skins.

Arthropods were probably able to acquire blood meals from dinosaurs in antiquity. The barbed, saw like, hyperstome mouth of the tick may have evolved to pierce the thick hide of a dinosaur (Nuwer, 2014)! When humans came around, the ticks and the bacteria they harbor were already present and ready for blood meals and pathogen transfers.

Why did bacteria and ticks get together? Bacteria are naturally found in soil where they are vulnerable to the elements. Wind, rain, and even sunlight can have a detrimental effect. The tick and other arthropods, insects, and animals provide protection as well as a rich source of vital nutrients for vulnerable bacteria. For the tick, bacteria can act as symbionts. Genome analysis has found that symbionts provide their tick hosts with vitamins and co-factors. In addition to gut bacteria, about twenty percent of insect species harbor symbiotic bacteria called endocytobiotes. Many endosymbionts are associated with insects that live on unbalanced diets and they are essential for the persistence of these hosts in their particular ecological niches (primary symbionts) (Lehane, 1991). For several herbivorous insects, it has been proposed that symbiotic bacteria, including early *Bartonella* and *Rickettsia,* may have recycled nitrogenous waste products into usable amino acids (Anderson et al., 2012). They may help degrade urea into ammonia, which in turn can be converted into glutamine and glutamate. Urea derives from uric acid, the major waste product released by insects into the hindgut (McNally et al., 1965).

Bartonella evolved from an insect associated gut symbiont before it started its long association with cats! The blood meals taken by ticks and other vectors are lacking in B vitamins. Some symbiotic bacteria have the capacity to synthesize B vitamins to fill this deficiency (Le Blanc, et al., 2012). This may be the case for the *Borrelia* and *Ixodes* ticks, which have been associated for more than 15 million years, perhaps providing the ticks with the capability to feed exclusively on blood. A study of symbiont bacteria showed that much of their genome is devoted to vitamin synthesis. In lice, symbionts make B-vitamins.

In contrast to those of free-living bacteria, the genome of *Borrelia* is relatively small, probably reflecting its lifestyle as an

obligate parasite. *Borrelia* lack the conventionally recognizable machinery for synthesizing nucleotides, amino acids, fatty acids, and enzyme cofactors, apparently scavenging these necessities from their hosts.

Tick and mammalian hosts provide contrasting environments for bacterial growth. Notably, mammals regulate their body temperatures at about ninety eight degrees, whereas ticks vary with the ambient temperature, except when feeding on a mammal. Also, the pH of mammalian tissue and blood is neutral, whereas the tick midgut is a more acidic environment. In order to cycle between two very different hosts, *Borrelia* has evolved to vary its gene expression, leading to different protein components and enabling physiological adaptation to both environments.

Borrelia burgdorferi colonization increases the expression of several tick gut genes including pixr, encoding a secreted gut protein which plays a role in larval molting. Although the functions of only a few *Borrelia burgdorferi* products have been clearly defined, some (such as OspC) are required for the bacteria to survive the initial attack of a mammalian Innate Immune System, while others (like VlsE) contribute to resisting the subsequent Acquired Immune response (Paulsen, et al, 2000).

The human body is in many ways a large set of symbiotic entities. Benign bacteria are protected and, in the course of their existence, provide services essential to human life-especially in the process of digesting food. Other bacteria, however, are either benign or harmful to human life. They can cause disease. The bacteria that ticks carry are "very opportunistic" write George Poinar, Jr., the world leading expert in amber analysis. "In the United States, Europe and Asia ticks carry bacteria that cause a wide range of diseases, affect many animal species, and often are not understood recognized by doctors. It's likely that many ailments in human history for which doctors had no explanation have been caused by tick-borne disease. Lyme Disease is a perfect example. It can cause problems with joints, the heart and central nervous system, but researchers didn't even know it existed until 1975. As long as humans have been around, I'm sure that they have suffered from ailments caused by spirochetes carried by ticks

(Nuwer, 2014). Dr. Poinar's work shows that all of the elements necessary for the current Lyme Disease pandemic: trees, ticks, bacteria and blood meal hosts were already in place millions of years before humans walked the earth

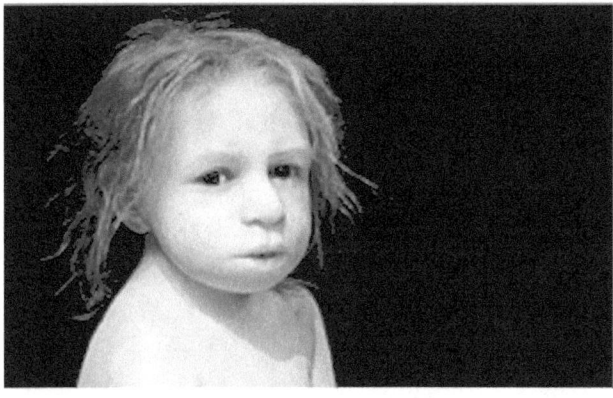

Figure 25. A reconstruction of a 'Neanderthal child.' Museum at Les Eyzies-de-Tayac, France. Photo credit: AP.

NANDY: THE NEANDERTHAL WITHIN US

The Neanderthals were an Archaic Human species that lived in or near the deciduous forests of Europe and Central Asia for over five hundred thousand years before they became extinct. They may be gone, but some of their genes are very much alive within many modern humans. Recent DNA findings are beginning to transform our understanding of positive selection in humans, both by introducing the concept of the adaptive introgression of archaic DNA into the human genome and by showing that any analysis of past genetics that is based upon present-day populations creates unreliable models. Some widely held hypotheses about the effects of selective forces are also beginning to seem unreliable.

Analysis of DNA from Mesolithic Europeans shows that adaptive variants associated with pathogen resistance were already present in our hunter-gatherers ancestors long before the advent of agriculture and that some were even inherited from the Neanderthals. Even lactose tolerance, which was assumed to have been selected for by participants in the Agricultural Revolution, appears to have been an absent trait among most early European farmers. Dairy intake among humans increased dramatically in just

the past three thousand years, but it took the arrival of the almost forgotten Yamnaya for it to happen in Europe. Ancient genomes can inform our understanding of the history of human adaptation through the direct tracking of changes in genetic variant frequency across different geographical locations and time periods. Our story, including the history of human interaction with Lyme disease, starts with a trip back about eighty thousand years at the time when Early Modern Humans met their distant Neanderthal and Denisovan Archaic Human relatives for the first time.

Most of today's Modern Humans outside of African, and even some in Africa, have just a bit of measurable archaic human DNA but what they have packs a powerful punch. A whopping fifty percent of the components of our immune systems are inherited from the Archaics. This inheritance helped the human race survive but it also comes with a few drawbacks. A gene mutation, for example, which increases the modern risk for arthritis seems to have evolved during the Ice Ages to help protect our ancestors from frostbite. Around half of all modern Europeans carry the variant of the GDF5 gene which nearly doubles their chance of developing painful joints, and also knocks a tiny bit off their adult height (Capellini, et al, 2016).

Before his body came to rest permanently in the Shalimar Cave, the Neanderthal man that has been nicknamed "Nandy"by his archaeological excavators, was a short fellow who had lived the hard knock life of a Neanderthal. This cave site, dating from between 60-80,000 years BP, produced nine skeletons of Neanderthals of varying ages, states of preservation, and degree of completeness. When he died Nandy was an old Neanderthal male who displayed a mosaic of health problems and deformities. He was aged between 40-50 years old and had trauma-related abnormalities, which is his case would have been debilitating to the point of making day-to-day life painful. At some point in his life he had suffered a violent blow to the left side of his face, creating a crushing fracture to his left orbit which would have left him partially or totally blind in one eye. He also suffered from a withered right arm which had been fractured in several places and healed, but which caused the loss of his lower arm and hand. This

could have been congenital, the result of childhood disease and trauma, or due to an amputation later in his life. His arm had healed but he may have had some paralysis down his right side, leading to deformities in his lower legs and foot, which would have resulted in him walking with a pronounced, painful limp (Trinkaus et al., 1982, 61).

All these injuries were acquired long before death, showed extensive healing, with little or no sign of infection and are evidence that Neanderthals cared for their sick, injured and elderly, prolonging their lives and making allowances for injuries and illnesses that would have left them as burdens on the social group (Dettwyler, 1991, 379). A Neanderthal skeleton, that is referred to as an "old man" from La Chapelle, France, shows joint degeneration or arthritis on his mandible (Cave and Strauss, 1957). Another individual suffered from a degenerative joint disorder in his foot, which would have resulted in painful, limited movement. Quite old by the time he died, bone had re-grown along the gums where he had lost several teeth, perhaps decades before. In fact, he lacked so many teeth that it's possible he needed his food ground down before he was able to eat it. Other Neanderthals in his social group may have supported him in his final years as he suffered from "gross deforming osteoarthritis"(Trinkaus, 1982).

Within the West Asian and European record there are five broad groups of pathology or injury noted in Neanderthal skeletons: fractures, trauma, degenerative diseases, hypoplastic diseases and infections. The high frequency of fractures and trauma seen in a greater degree of Neanderthals suggest that they had a different and more dangerous spear driven hunting style (Klein, 1999, 475) than other human groups. They may have been much more 'up close and personal' with hunted animals which added more wear and tear on the Neanderthal body and increased the risk of tick-borne infections.

Evidence of infections on Neanderthal skeletons are most visible in the form of lesions of the bone. Archaic skeletons have been found with evidence of degenerative lesions on femors, tibias and fibulas, indicative of a systemic infection like *Borrelia* and/or carcinoma (malignant tumor/cancer). Arthritis seems to have been

very common in the older Neanderthal population, specifically targeting areas of articulation such as the knees, ankle (Shanidar III), spine and hips (La Chapelle-aux-Saints 'Old Man'), arms (La Quina, Krapina, Feldhofer), fingers and toes. Degenerative joint disease, which can range from normal, use-related degeneration to painful, debilitating restriction of movement and deformity is seen in varying degree in all the Shanidar skeletons (Solecki & Agelarakis, 2004).

Neanderthals seem to have been knowledgeable about natural medicines to fight pain and infection. One rather sick Neanderthal from a site at El Sidrón[Spain] was eating a steady diet of poplar, the bark of which contains the painkiller salicylic acid- the active ingredient in aspirin, as well as plants that were covered in *Penicillium* mold, which generates the famous antibiotic. Yarrow, Cornflower, Bachelor's Button, St. Barnaby's Thistle, Ragwort or Groundsel, Grape Hyacinth, Joint Pine or Woody Horsetail and Hollyhock have been found in association with one Neanderthal grave, all of which have long-known medicinal properties as diuretics, stimulants, and astringents as well as anti-inflammatory properties (Solecki, 1975, 881).

The Neanderthal confronted a variety of pathogens, including *Borrelia*. As Hunter-Gatherers in post-glacial temperate deciduous forests they would have been at a high risk for tick borne infections. *Borrelia* seem to have gotten into their bones. Neanderthals, like all hunter-gatherer groups, had a high rate of bone infections.The proclivity of Neanderthal Toll Like Receptors for attacking viruses shows that they also confronted them all those years ago. They certainly experienced a whole set of *retrovirouses*, which are so ancient that some of them have actually become fused into our human genome. These ancient viruses have persistently infected humans at very low levels for hundreds of thousands or even millions of years. The *retrovirus* is a kind of living fossil. It replicates by inserting its genome into an infected cell. Occasionally, *retroviruses* infect 'germ line' cells – eggs and sperm – and if these cells create a new organism, that new organism will contain the *retrovirus* as an inherent part of its genome.

In this way, the genomes of many mammals, birds and other vertebrates have accumulated DNA sequences derived from *retroviruses*, known as endogenous *retroviruses* [ERVs]. About eight percent of the modern human genome is comprised of ERVs. Some ERVs have been co-opted to perform physiological functions within host organisms-including providing a level of immunity. Some of these viruses cause asymptomatic infections, some are known for causing persistent infections resulting in slow but progressive disease, and some cause lifelong infections. Although it has a modern genesis, the most well known of the type of *retrovirus* is Human Immunodeficiency Virus [HIV], which causes Acquired Immune Deficiency Syndrome [AIDS].

Before Early Modern Humans arrived in Eurasia, the Neanderthal immune system would already have had a lot of experience with a plethora of pathogens. *Retroviruses,* bacteria, and other infections circulated within a climate that, unlike Africa, included a cold winter season. Newly arrived Early Modern Humans had immune systems that had developed in year round warmth that incubated a different set of pathogens. To survive in different climates, both groups had developed different Innate Immune Systems that could be best described as rapid response teams.

At first blush, African immunity was not well suited to the pathogens that were thriving in the new climate, while the Neanderthals and Denisovans that they interacted with had immune systems that were no longer experienced with African incubated infections. When our human ancestors mated with Neanderthals all those years ago, they exchanged disease-related genes as well as pathogens. Diseases passed on to Neanderthals. Infections likely to have been passed include tapeworm, tuberculosis, herpes and other viruses and *Helicobacter pylori,* a strain of bacteria that causes stomach ulcers. It infected humans for the first time in Africa at least 88,000 years ago and first arrived in Europe about 52,000 years ago (Houldcroft & Underdown, 2016).

Even though Neanderthals and Denisovans eventually became extinct, humans went on to populate the modern world with an entire assemblage of associated fauna and pathogens, and a

hybrid set of immune responses.

Neanderthals, having already lived in Europe for thousands of years, had coped with the risk of bacterial sepsis by evolving a strong Interleukin 18 [IL18] gene that plays a central role in the Innate Immune System. Decreased levels produced by introgressed genes are protective for risk of infection. Another introgressed allele, a truncated form of the OAS2 protein, alleviates symptoms of tick borne encephalitis [TBEV] in Europeans. TBEV is found in forested areas of north, central, and eastern Europe, which would have formed a major part of the Neanderthal's typical ecosystem. Neanderthal introverted TLR's have a higher expression in response to Epstein Barr Viruses ((Houldcroft & Underdown, 2016)

Ironically, it may have been the close personal contact that also doomed the Archaics. All of the mosquito associated viruses that circulate in Europe, Asia, Australia and/or the Americas, appear to have evolutionary roots in Africa. The *Flaviviridae* family includes several tick-borne viruses that affect humans. The Old World diversity of *flaviviruses* and the comparatively lower number of New World viruses make an 'Out-of-Africa' history seem to be the most plausible interpretation for *flavivirus* phylogenetic distribution.

Flaviviruses are the new kids on the virus block. DNA studies have found that *flavivirus* originated between about 85,000 and 120,000 years ago (Petterson & Fiz-Palacios, 2014). All major tick- borne *flavivirus* clades contain African viruses (Chambers & Monath, 2003). With this dating, it is quite likely that the *flaviviruses* were carried into Europe, Asia, and North America in association with the waves of human migration that began at some point after between 125,000 and 60,000 years ago. The *flavivirus* Tick-borne Encephalitis (TBEV) was first identified in 1932 as a severe neurological disease that occurred in forest workers in the far eastern Soviet Union (now Russia). In 1936 an exploratory expedition found that *Ixodes persulcatus* was the vector for TBEV. In 1937, individual groups identified the causative agent of TBE to be a virus that was subsequently called "far-eastern encephalitis virus" (Zlobin, et al, 2017).

Powassan Virus is another ancient *flavivirus* that has also been recently "discovered" by modern medicine. It is tick-borne *(Brackney, et al. 2008)* and affects humans in North America (Ebel, et al 2001). It is named after the town of Powassan, Ontario, Canada, where it was first identified in 1958 (McLean, et al 1959). The virus is found in a temperate zone across Eurasia, where it is part of the tick borne encephalitis-complex (Subbotina and Loktev, 2012). It appears to be currently spreading in the United States and Canada. Small and medium-sized mammals act as reservoirs including woodchucks [*Marmota monax*] and white-footed mice [*Peromyscus leucopus*]) and several species of tick, including *Ixodes,* are the vectors. *Powassan* was probably introduced into North America some time between the opening and closing of the Bering Strait land bridge that connected with Asia between 15,000 and 11,000 years ago (Hikar,et al, 2011, Weyrauch, 2017)

European territory was not populated by Early Modern Humans until after 45,000 years ago (except for some southernrefuges), was depopulated during the Last Glacial Maximum that began 25,000 years ago, and subsequently was repopulated only after the climate improved. Groups that left behind skeletons that appear to combine human and Neanderthal features are found to date from the post-glacial time period. Humans with Neanderthal introgressed immune systems would have had the advantage of inheriting immune systems experienced in fighting both European and African pathogens.

We are all descendants of people who lived to an age where they could reproduce and have immune systems that have been been sorted and refined by waves of experiences with disease. Some epidemics killed off swaths of people. Some of these disease cataclysms are known from historical records and others can only be found through research within a variety of disciplines. Plague, smallpox, influenza, AIDS and other earlier unknown pathogens have played a role in shaping human immunity and demographics. There have been several times in the past when human populations in specific geographic areas on the earth have been completely replaced by other human populations. This appears to have

happened to the Neanderthal, who had little experience fighting *flavivirus* and went extinct after it was brought out of Africa.

Demic diffusion is a migratory model, developed by Luigi Luca Cavalli-Sforza, of population spreading into and across an area that had been previously uninhabited by that group, possibly, but not necessarily displacing, replacing, or intermixing with a pre-existing population. This may be related to warfare, but pathogens seem to play a central role in the history of diffusion (Cavalli-Sforza & Mench, 1997).

After the extinction of the Neanderthal, Europe was repopulated by three subsequent migrations. The demic diffusion model for Europe required a substantial revision after the DNA of several 7,000 to 8,000-year-old individuals from Western Europe and a 24,000-year-old individual from Siberia showed that three different ancient populations have contributed to the genetics of present-day Europeans: (1) West European hunter-gatherers, (2) Early European farmers, who were mainly of Middle Eastern origin and (3) overwhelmingly Ancient Northern Eurasians (Gibbons, 2014).

All carried a Neanderthal genes.The refined model shows that Mesolithic hunter-gatherers were affected by the arrival of farmers from the Middle East during the Early Neolithic. There was a major population turnover in Europe 14,500 years ago which eliminated mtDNA lineage M (Posth, et al, 2016). DNA samples of male European Hunter-Gatherers after this death event carried male Y haplogroups G2a, I, and occasionally F. I (particularly I2) was predominant while mtDNA haplogroup U (especially U5) was predominant for women. There was then a massive migration from the Eurasian Steppes at about 4,500 years ago by Y-haplotype R1a and R1b migrants of the Yamnaya culture. The genetic impact of the Yamnaya migration on the modern European and West Asian population is striking. G2a and F Y haplotypes are rare in present day Europe. Y haplogroups I1 and I2a1 have only a twenty percent rate in the present-day populations of Europe, with the highest frequencies in Scandinavia (Chikhi, 2002).

Ötzi [the ice mummy] had the Y haplotype G2a, which was part of a subhaplogroup that was frequent in the Neolithic

populations across Europe. The most characteristic mtDNA haplogroup of early farmers from the Carpathian Basin and Central Europe is N1a but there is a diversity of mtDNA haplogroups T2, J, K, HV, V, W and X, which are known as the mitochondrial 'Neolithic package' in Europe by 6,000 BC. When Agriculture that originated in the Fertile Crescent spread to Central Europe via the western Carpathian Basin: a geographic landscape that acted as a natural corridor and adaptation zone, it came with migrants. The Agricultural Revolution was genetic as well as cultural (Ammerman, A. J. & Cavalli-Sforza, L. L.,1984). It was also a fusion event. Hunter-gatherers contributed, on average ,thirty percent of the DNA in early agricultural settlements.

The diversity in mtDNA with the homogenity of Y-DNA among European Neolithic populations may illuminate early European social structure. Women seem to move around more than men. One plausible explanation for this phenomenon is patrilocality (where women move to their husband's birth place after the marriage). Other possibilities that could lead to similar observations include polygamy or male-biased adult mortality. A patrilocal residential rule was possibly linked to a system of descent along the father's line (patrilineality) in early farming communities.

Ethnographic studies have suggested a change of residential rules at the advent of the Neolithic, showing different trends in residential rules among foragers and non-foragers. Increasing sedentism promoted territorial defense and control of resources, favoring men in the inheritance of land and property, which consequently led to patrilocal residence. While patrilocality might have caused high mtDNA diversity within populations, observations from many sites in Europe argue for a common set of cultural and social practices across large distances for early farming cultures in Europe that must have been spread largely by women (Szécsényi-Nagy, et al., 2015).

The dating of teeth found in China provides evidence of an early migration of Early Modern Humans from Africa into Southeast Asia at before 80,000-120,000 years ago (Dennell, 2015). A later major migration from Africa traveled along the coast

of Arabia and Persia to India and the rest of South Asia. Along the way Early Modern Humans interbred with both Neanderthals and Denisovans (Dennell, R. & Petraglia, M. 2012).

It appears that Lyme disease exposure differed between various groups of early humans, especially during the Last Glacial Maxima when isolated human populations retreated to refuges. One was in the grassy Eurasian steppes. Another was East Asia in an area of temperate forest. The ice cut the East Asians off from the Central Asians, who were also isolated from people refuging in what is now Southern France and Spain. As small genetic mutations accumulated, various ethnically-associated characteristics began to develop. These included Innate Immune Systems with varying experiences with tick-borne disease, especially B*orrelia*. Physical traits that were appropriate to specific environments developed through specific epigenetic processes (Szécsényi-Nagy, 2015).

Importantly, experienced infections changed our genes. Immune system genetics that did a good job at fighting off whatever was thrown at it have survived. One of the worst epidemics known to humanity came in the form of a flea bite-the Black Death or plague-and actually changed our genes. By comparing an Eastern European genome to that of a Roma population that lived in the same territory since before 1300 AD with a group of Roma from India that had never encountered the plague, they found that Europeans and Roma had shared alterations to their genetic code that occurred in the Roma after they settled in Europe. They found almost twenty genes that showed evidence of convergent evolution, meaning that the two groups started out different but evolved similarly because of shared pressures from their shared environment.

One involved gene, SLC45A2, which is known to be involved in skin pigmentation, points to an important role for Vitamin D in fighting disease. Others are linked to immune-system function. The immune-related cluster, called Toll Like Receptor 2, is known to help immune cells recognize and destroy foreign invaders. The Black Death put strong pressure on this gene cluster to evolve. Some TLR2 variations got weeded out. When

researchers looked at how TLR2 reacted to *Yersinia pestis* and *Yersinia pseudo tuberculosis,* the shared form of TLR2 caused a heightened immune response. They found that humans have been modified, basically, by infections (Laayouni, et al, 2014). How our immune system reacts to *Borrelia* and other infections is strongly linked to our ancestral experiences.

TABLE 3.   NEANDERTHAL DISEASE PACKAGES

PLEISTOCENE

BACTERIA

Borrelia, Brucellosis, Heliobacter pylori, Leperosy, Tuberculosis,Streptococcuus mutans, Pertusis, Salmonella typhi, Staphylococci,Tuleraemia, Yaws

PARASITES

Lice, **Ticks**, Pinworms, Tapeworms, Whipworms

VIRUSES

Adenoviruses, Coronaviridae, Flaviviruses, Hepatitis A, Herpesviridae, HPV, Polyomaviridae, Rhabdoviridae

EARLY HOLOCENE

BACTERIA

Cholera, Diphtheria, Leptospirosis, Neisseria gonorrhoea, Yersinia pestis,

PARASITES

Helminths, Plasmodium vivax, Plasmodium falciparum

VIRUSES

Norovirus, Hepatitus B,C & E, HIV, HTLV, Infuenza, Lymphocytic chorionic meningitis, Measles, Mumps

Neanderthal Infectious Disease Genetics from Houldcroft & Underdown, 2016.

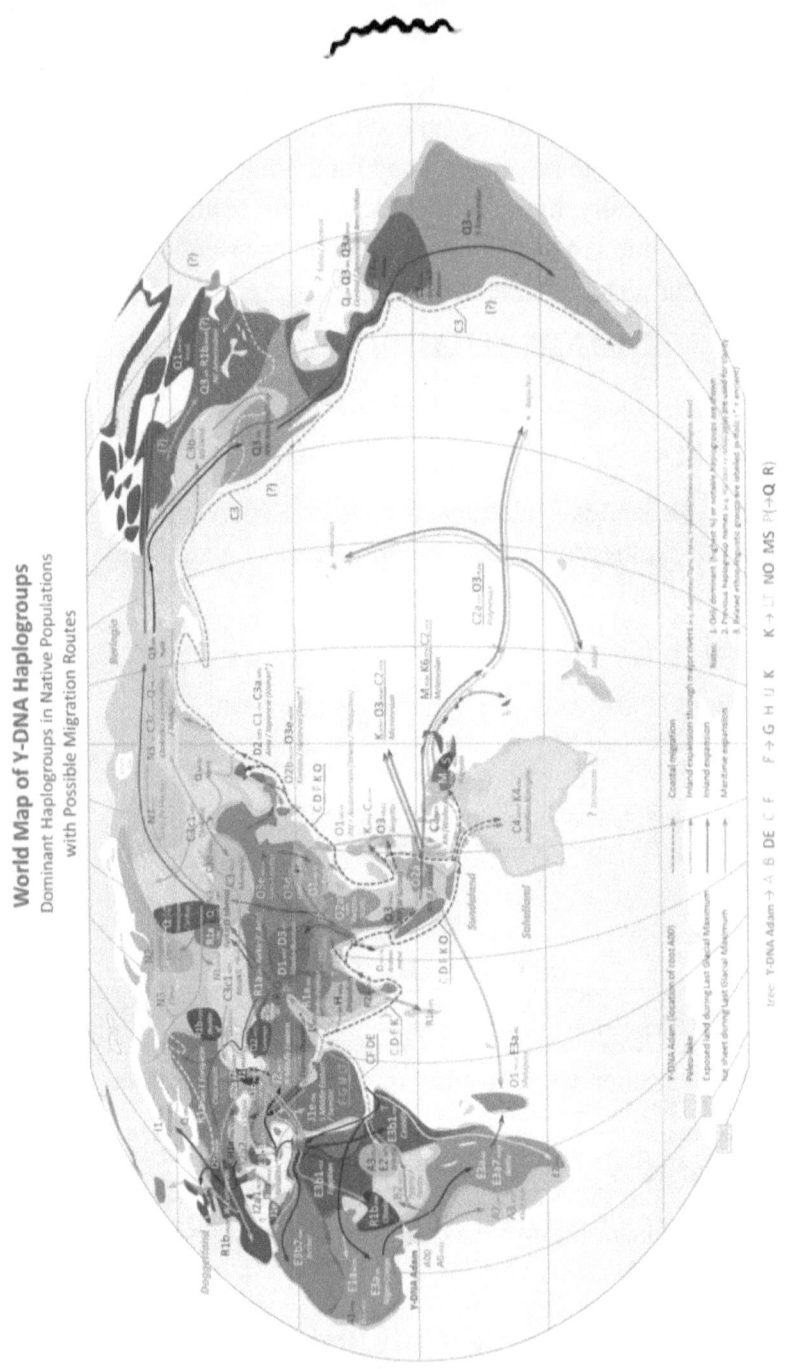

Figure 26. Chakazul, Infographics, Creative Commons

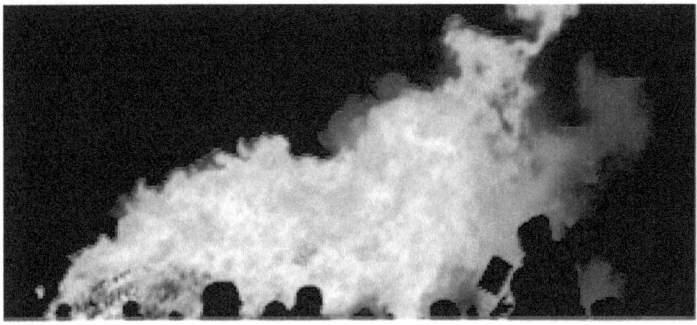

Figure 27. The bonfire originally was originally fueled by bones and wood. http://esol.britishcouncil.org.

THE HAND OF MAN: LANDSCAPES ON FIRE

The controlled use of fire is one of the earliest of human discoveries. It may have facilitated human evolution. Fire has been used to add light and heat, to cook food, to clear forests for grazing and planting, to harden stone, to melt metals to create tools and other objects, to keep predators away, to fire clay for ceramic objects, and most importantly for this volume, to kill vermin and sanitize pathogens. Fires have social purposes as well- as gathering places, as messages or beacons, to mark special events and as spaces for important activities. The control of fire was probably a staged process: opportunistic use of fire from natural occurrence followed by limited conservation and maintenance of fires lit by natural occurrences in wet or cold seasons; and finally, the mastery of the ability to kindle or create fire (Gowlett, 2016).

The controlled use of fire probably occurred during the Paleolithic Age. The earliest evidence for fire associated with humans comes from the Oldwan sites in the Lake Turkana region of Kenya. The site of Koobi Fora (dated 1.6 million years ago) contains oxidized patches of earth to a depth of several centimeters, which some archeologists interpret as evidence for controlled fire. At 1.4 million years of age, the

Australopithecus site at Chesowanja in central Kenya also contained burned clay clasts in small areas. Lower Paleolithic sites in Africa with evidence for fire include Gadeb in Ethiopia (burned rock), Swartkrans (270 burned bones, dated 600,000-1 million years old) and Wonderwerk Cave (burned ash and bone fragments, ca. 1 million years ago), both in South Africa (Gowlett & Wrangham, 2013).

The earliest evidence for controlled use of fire outside of Africa is at the Lower Paleolithic site of Gesher Benot Ya'aqov in Israel, where charred wood and seeds were recovered from a site dated to 790,000 years ago. The next oldest site is at Zhoukoudian, a Lower Paleolithic site in China and Beeches Pit in the UK, both at about 400,000 years ago, and at Qesem Cave (Israel), between about 200,000-400,000 years ago. Habitual use of fire was firmly established by about 400,000 years ago (Twomey, 2013), but may have occurred earlier based upon the appearance of fire pits, changes in settlement patterns and physical traits like human brain size and changes towards a smaller mouth, teeth and digestive systems. The adoption of cooking, which softens food and makes it easier to digest, could have led to these changes (Gowlett & Wrangham, 2013).

The control of fire enabled important changes in human behavior, health, energy expenditure, and geographic expansion. As a result of "domesticating" fire, hominids were able to modify their environments to their own benefit. This ability to manipulate environments allowed them to move into much colder regions that would have previously been uninhabitable after the loss of body hair. There is evidence that suggests that fire was used to clear out caves prior to living in them. Early hominids used grass fires to hunt and to control the population of pests in the surrounding area (Bellomo, 1994). The Neanderthals may even have frequently burned their bedding to eliminate parasites (Kuhn, 2009). Burning and animal grazing, if intensive enough, would have thinned and ultimately eliminated forest in some areas (Herculano-Houzel, 2016).

Both "push" and "pull" factors may have prompted Early Modern Humans to leave Africa and colonize Eurasia in a

staggered manner. The Middle Eastern Levant of 100,000 to 150,000 years ago was essentially an extension of northeastern Africa and was probably part of the original range of hominids. Temperature and aridity data from the Horn of Africa region suggest that warm and wet conditions from 120,000 to 90,000 years ago would have facilitated early waves of human migration toward the Levant and Arabia, which is supported by fossil and lithic evidence. However, the primary Out-of-Africa event occurred during a cold and dry time. At around 70,000 years ago, climate in the Horn of Africa shifted from a wet phase called "Green Sahara" to even drier than the region is now. The region also became colder. Researchers analyzed ancient leaf wax in sediment deposits that showed that the time people migrated out of Africa coincided with a big shift to a much drier and colder climate suggesting a drought everywhere in northeast Africa. Genetic research indicates that a large group of people migrated from Africa into Eurasia between 70,000 and 55,000 years ago (Tierney and Zander, 2017).

  This wave of *homo sapiens* reproduced rapidly, and settled the Middle East; smaller groups went off to India and China. Isolated by mountains and the sea for many generations, and exposed to a colder climate and less sunlight than in Africa, the Asian populations became paler. Around 40,000 years ago, when the grip of the Ice Age loosened and temperatures briefly became warmer, humans moved up into Central Asia. Amid the bountiful grassy steppes, they multiplied quickly. Some have said, "If Africa was the cradle of mankind, then Central Asia was its nursery" (Wells, 2004).

  Around 35,000 years ago, small groups left Central Asia for Europe. Cut off from other people, these migrants became paler and shorter than their African ancestors. From there, around 20,000 years ago, another small group of Central Asians moved farther north into Siberia and the Arctic Circle. As they moved around, they traversed landscapes with varying levels of risk for interactions with the *Ixodes* ticks and *Borrelia*. Interactions within grassland and pine forests would have been safe, while forays into temperate deciduous forests would have been highly risky, based

on modern landscape studies (Elton, 2008). Our ancestors confronted these risks with fire!

Tick presence in the North Central United States has been positively associated with deciduous dry/mesic and dry forests, fertile soils such as alfisols, sand and loamy/sand soil texture, and sedimentary bedrock. There was a negative association with grasslands and conifer forests, wet and wet/mesic forests, acidic soils such as spodosols, clay soil texture, and Precambrian bedrock. Elevation was not an important discriminator in the model (Guerra, M., et al., March 2002).

One of the most useful tools for modern Lyme disease epidemiologists has been the Geographic Information System (hereafter GIS). Using a Landsat Thematic Mapper, various elements can be factored into satellite geological system generated risk maps to predict the presence of the optimum tick vectors. This type of analysis is slated to be undertaken in New England, U.S.A. in the future because the incidence of Lyme disease is on the rise in that area. It has been done very effectively in Westchester County, New York, a Lyme disease endemic area. Information from the ground, developed through drag sampling and canine serology reports was compared and correlated with the satellite generated GIS map data for risk.

In a study of three hundred and thirty seven residential properties, high-risk properties consistently tested as being both significantly greener than low risk properties. High-risk properties appeared to contain a greater proportion of broadleaf trees, while low risk properties had more non-vegetative cover and open grassy lawn. The model that was developed was then tested further by comparing it with data about human infection that was obtained through a random questionnaire that was sent out to property owners in the area. By comparing predicted with observed (questionnaire responses) data, a seventy one percent accuracy was found for the remote sensory prediction of risk(Nicholson & Mather,1994). Another study, also done in Westchester County, used canine seroprevalence rates to analyze the effect of residential adjacency to forest on Lyme disease risk. This study found that the rate of Lyme infected dogs was positively correlated

with living adjacent to the forest (Beck, 2000).

A study done in Maryland used ground-based zip codes to map annual risk for Lyme disease. It found that the greatest risk areas for actual infection occurred along green riparian features, especially along the watershed areas. This was well correlated with a GIS assessment for the area. These riparian zones were regularly used by deer and other wildlife as a source of drinking water (Frank, et al, 2002). Another study done in Maryland concluded that contact between humans, ticks, and wildlife vector hosts is facilitated in landscapes with high forest-herbaceous interspersion or edge environments. Both deer and field mice thrive in these heterogeneous landscapes. Deer prefer a mix of forest cover and open areas with tender grassy vegetation. The mouse is highly opportunistic and will inhabit both forest edges and open patches (Jackson, 2005).

All of these habitats may, by coincidence, be adjacent to human habitation areas and Lyme disease is strongly associated with peri-domestic exposure. This spatial pattern is most likely to occur in a modern suburban setting and historically in a landscape featuring a dispersed settlement pattern within dense deciduous forest.

While both masting and moisture levels play important roles in Lyme disease infection rates, land cover patterns are also significant features for these infections. In one study, Lyme disease rates were found to be highest where there was the greatest amount of edge interspersion between grassy lawn and forest, with a ratio that included forty to sixty percent herbaceous cover. The analyzed spatial characteristics plot as being high risk or low risk (Jackson, et al.,2005).

Archaic and Early Modern humans lived in a variety of landscapes. Over time, some human populations left the grassy savannas and headed north into the tick risky landscapes of Eurasia with a low-density, mobile, hunting and gathering life-style that interacted with a new mosaic of grasslands and dense forests. Eventually most groups, including the pastoralists of the Eurasian Steppes, changed to a communal living pattern where they interacted with the heavily modified landscapes of agricultural

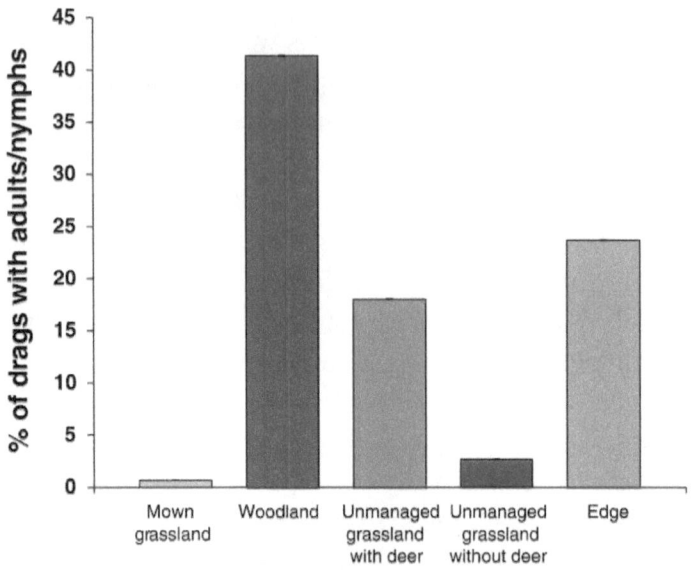

Figure 28. Percentage of drags with adult or nymphal *Ixodes ricinus* ticks in each different habitat type surveyed. Grassland harbors few ticks.(Jennett, A., Smith, F.& Wall, R., 2013).

pastures and settlements. This new, man-made environment had both rewards and risks. While being inherently less tick risky, there was an uptick in the growth of mosquitos. Cleared land led to numerous small water collections close to human habitation areas. The mosquito population increased because of access to stable and accessible sources of blood in the human population, leading to an increased spread of vectors of malaria, especially in Africa and the Mediterranean basin (Carter & Mendis, 2002).

Even though the practice of agriculture developed throughout the tropics and subtropics of Asia and the Middle East up to several thousand years before it spread to Africa, simultaneous animal domestication in Asia probably prevented mosquitoes from feeding exclusively on humans. In most parts of the world, the probability

of a blood meal being on a human for the vectors of malaria is much less than fifty percent and often less than ten to twenty percent, but in sub-Saharan Africa, it is eighty to almost one hundred percent. This is probably the most important single factor responsible for the stability and intensity of malaria transmission in tropical Africa (Elton, 2008).

For *Ixodes* ticks, humans are an incidental blood meal host but Lyme disease has been an omnipresent risk, with flares and pockets of infection, for millennia. Regular interaction with tick-risky environments resulted in infection. Various bio-archeological studies have found that Hunter-Gatherers had higher rates of arthritic-type joint infections than Agriculturalists, which may be related to their frequent contact with tick risky forested areas. People living in the Age of Industrialization, in one study, had the lowest arthritis rates of all, while modern suburban populations, especially since the middle of the twentieth century, have exceeded rates for all other time periods by a large margin.

A study of degenerative joint disease of the major appendicular joints in hunter-gatherers and agriculturalists from northwestern Alabama found that shoulders, elbows, and knees were more likely to be infected than the hip and ankle. There are virtually no sex differences in the hunter-gatherer group, but among agriculturalists, males had more severe osteoarthritis than females. The hunters-gatherers had a slightly greater prevalence of arthritis than the agriculturalists (Bridges,1991). In general, the switch to a settled agricultural lifestyle made people shorter and sicker but prevented arthritis (Ross, 2011, Mummert, et al, 2011). Arthritis came roaring back in the trunk of a car. It is associated with the car centric suburbanization movement of the twentieth century, which moved people out next to a forest full of deer that were no longer being hunted.

The modern map of Lyme disease risk in the United States is heavily focused in the New England and Mid Atlantic area. In the modern landscape, a particular set of biological and environmental circumstances has converged to create the perfect storm of conditions for the modern Lyme disease outbreak. Forest has returned to land that was cleared for farming and dispersed

suburban neighborhoods have developed. There is now more forest in many places in New England, for example, than at any time in the previous one hundred and fifty years.

This secondary forest occurs patchily amid occupied spaces creating an edge habitat, which is ideal for deer and ticks. The deer population has exploded because wolves were hunted to extinction leaving no remaining natural predators in New England. Hunting is restricted in suburban living areas. Americans became exposed to Lyme disease in the twentieth century when they moved en masse into the deer/tick habitat of the suburb. A similar story occurred in the growing suburbs of Europe and Asia (Foster, 2005). It appears that Lyme disease exposure differed between various groups of early humans. Africa has a few small pockets of *Borrelia* but most of the risk is in Eurasia and North America, dependent on landscape and habitat.

While refuged from the Last Glacial Maxima, physical traits appropriate to specific environments developed in isolated groups of humans. At around 15,000 years ago, as the last Ice Age began to wane, one small clan of Arctic dwellers followed a reindeer herd over the Bering Strait land bridge into North America. According to the genetic data this initial group may have included as few as two or three men-perhaps only ten to twenty people in all. Once isolated in the Americas, they too began to acquire distinct physical characteristics (Wells, 2004).

Archaeological and genetic data suggest that the source populations of modern humans that survived the glacial maximas and that human Y-DNA haplogroups emerged from sparsely refugia, and dispersed through a landscape of high primary productivity while avoiding dense forest cover (Gavashewithin lishvili & Tarkhnishvili, 2016). This may be related to the use of fire. Purposeful use of fire is tied to the burning of wood. Purposeful selection of wood fuel was a learned behavior: hardwood like oak burns differently from softwood- the moisture content and density of a wood all affect how hot or how long a fire burns. Other fuel sources became important in places with limited wood supply. Alternative fuels such as peat, cut turf, animal dung, bones, seaweed, and straw and hay can be used in a fire.

In a recent study, the researchers combined analyses of Ice Age accumulations of silt with computer simulations to formulate new interpretations of archaeological data. Some previous reconstructions of vegetation based on pollen and plant remains from lakes and marshland have suggested that Europe had an open steppe vegetation. But new computer simulations based on eight possible climate scenarios show that under natural conditions the landscape in large areas of Europe would have been far more densely forested that it actually was. The researchers conclude that human activity must have been responsible for the difference. Further evidence comes from traces of the use of fire in hunting settlements from this period and in the layers of ash found in the soil (Kalan, et al, 2016).

    Landscape clearing processes continued unabated during the late Neolithic into the early Bronze Ages. Charcoal layers and successive decreases in forest pollens, followed by increases in cereal and weed pollens in peat deposits, interbedded with farming and clearing implements, leave one in no doubt about the sequence of forest clearing (Williams, 2000). The cumulative effect of human wood use on the earth's forests, especially in cooler northern areas has been so pervasive and so great that the concept of a virgin forest has been "a fiction" since the Neolithic. Rather it was a "cultural landscape" in which " all vegetation types were created or modified by man." (Cronon, 2003). The story is similar for tropical forests.

    The first sedentary farmers in Europe—the Neolithic Agriculturalists—who began significant forest clearing and established permanent settlement from roughly 4,500 BP onwards were followed by the pastoralists from the steppes, who burned swaths of forest to open up grassy pasture for their herds of domesticated cattle, sheep, and horses. In Eastern North America, it was not until about 1,000 years ago that settlements began to diminish the vast continental forests, though the known impact was much earlier in South and Central America (Williams, 2008).

    Six thousand years ago, the landscape of Europe consisted

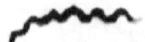

of densely forested areas with red deer feeding in closed habitats and early domesticated cattle grazing in more open landscapes. The forest was also a food resource for young cattle and pigs. This points to a great diversity of herding strategies and feeding techniques compared to later periods. The landscape was still rather forested, with no obvious changes in the habitat use of the large herbivores, five thousand years ago. However, carbon isotopes suggest a clearly reduced forest cover by four thousand years ago, with deer using similar open feeding grounds as domesticated cattle, based upon an analysis of the stable carbon isotope composition of archeological bone material from large herbivores showing paleo-environmental and vegetation changes, prehistoric animal management, and land-use (Doppler et al., 2015). Scientists have discovered that pottery was being made in China 20,000 year old, and fire eventually became commonly used to create pottery, which was more often than not used for the storage of agricultural products.(Bhanoo, June 28,2012).

Plague and war have had marked effect on forests. For example, after the Black Death epidemic of 1347 through 1353, between a fifth and a quarter of all settlements were abandoned across Europe. Studies of southern German pollen history show that the size of the forest increased (von Hoof, et al., 2006). Major European conflicts also reduced population and led to land abandonment and forest regrowth, notably the Hundred Years War (1337–1453), the Hussite wars in Bohemia (1419–36), the Wars of the Roses in England (1455-1485) and the devastating Thirty Years War, which was a veritable holocaust in central Europe between 1618 and 1648.

In the Americas,warfare was often associated with drought. After the introduction of European pathogens after 1492, there was a demographic collapse from a population of at least fifty three million to only five million by 1650, an 89 per cent decrease. Land abandonment was widespread and the forest increased in both extent and density. By 1750, North America was much more forested than it had been in 1492 (Denevan, 1992).

Prescribed burning on a regular basis has been an important part of human land management practices. They were part of the

slash and burn method of agricultural practice and were also part of European and Native American forest management programs. The typical regimen for applying prescribed burns was to do it on a regular basis as is verified by the archeological record. This "burning" was a regular activity that only could be disrupted by warfare, illness, or neglect.

Historically, Native Americans used fire to remove brush and undergrowth in forests and as a hunting strategy, though there's no evidence that they targeted ticks in the process. Many North American ecosystems are actually fire-dependent, meaning they need some occasional burning as part of their normal life cycles. Fires can occur naturally from lightning strikes, but since humans have already intervened in these ecosystems anyway, a prescribed burn can be a safe way of giving nature a helping hand. In some areas, the practice of prescribed burning still occurs and it is still quite common in the Southeast. The National Park Service reports that nearly sixty percent of its acres in the Southeast region are treated using prescribed burns (Geoffrey, 2016).

In other areas, especially in New England, fire use has declined. Burning does an excellent job of killing off *Ixodes* ticks and burning off the layer of accumulated leaf litter that ticks use as insulation against cold weather temperature. This effects both tick population levels and risk for tick borne infections. In one study, a 95.4 percent reduction in tick populations was found in areas that were regularly burned. This translated into an encounter with about one infected tick per every fifty hours spent in the geographical area. In contrast, someone walking through never-burned woods would cross paths with an infected tick every 1.5 hours. This translates to a ninety seven percent reduction in disease risk for regularly burned areas (Gleim, 2014).

In the United States the practice of burning off leaf litter and forest undergrowth has declined in recent decades. The decline began as our society industrialized and turned away from farming the land. Fire prevention campaigns like the ones using the character Smokey the Bear have made the public aware of the dangers of carelessness with fire. But they have also made people more reluctant to use fire responsibly as a tool for killing ticks. In

response to this, Smokey the Bear now warns against "wildfires," not all "forest fires," and the character's website describes the importance of controlled fires (Tripp, 2014). In New England, especially after the passage of The Clean Air Act in 1970, leaf burning in the fall and the burning off of the land in the spring decreased dramatically. Lyme disease was first identified in Lyme, Connecticut five years later in 1975 (Thomas, 2015).

The modern rise in tick-borne infection should be considered an unintended consequence or externality to this public policy. The history and benefit of prescribed fire have important implications for public health as it is an efficient, cost effective method for reducing tick populations and the risk of human tick-borne diseases.The use of fire as a tick control measure should be revisited by modern policy makers. Burn, baby, burn!

Effects of long-term burning on tick abundance at study plots

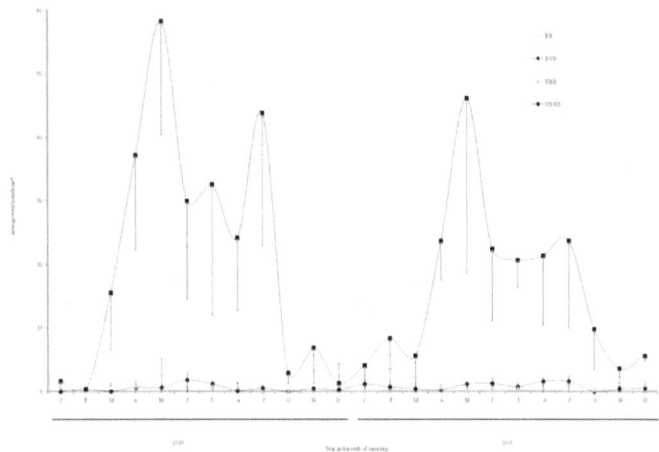

Figure 29. Modeling efforts suggested that total tick counts were affected by long-term burning, season, litter cover, and tree density. There was a significant interaction between burning and season. For plots in which burning occurred, tick counts did not change significantly by season [RR = 1.1 (95% CI: 0.57, 2.12); P=0.774], confirming the trend that ticks were significantly reduced in burned plots. However, at plots in which there was no burning, tick counts were 10 times greater in the warm season than in the cold [Relative Risk (RR) =10.7 (95% CI: 4.20, 27.18); P<0.001]. Having higher than 95% litter cover was positively associated with an approximately two-fold increase in tick counts and density of trees >183 per ha. was associated with an approximately six-fold increase in tick counts.Long-term prescribed burning significantly reduced tick counts. (Gleim, E.R., et al., November 6, 2014).

THE CRADLE OF LYME DISEASE?
BORRELIA IN THE BONE.

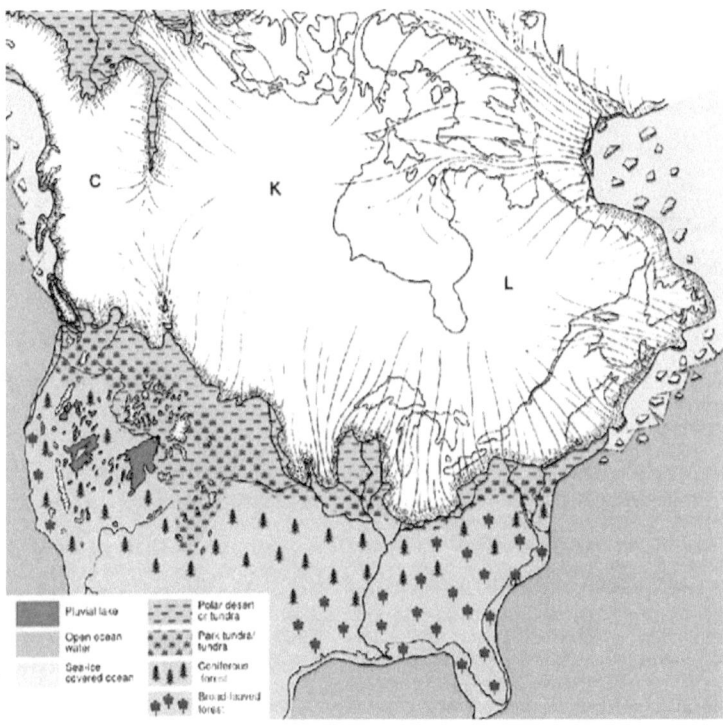

Figure 30. North America at 18000 BP. [Modern shorelines shown] Environmental ecotones moved up and down with the advance and retreat of glaciers. Note that the Temperate Broadleaf Forest that is GOOD habitat for *Ixodes* ticks was limited to two mixed zones on either side of the Proto-Mississippi River. As the glaciers melted, temperate forest moved northward. *Borrelia* were already present in North America long before humans arrived. When the earliest human occupants and their dogs walked or sailed across to North America they interacted with forested areas that had not yet been subjected to "the hand of man" and especially prescribed fire, which may have made these ancient migrants especially vulnerable to tick-borne infections. The tick risky forest edge was aligned with modern day Tennessee but slowly moved north over time. Hunter-gatherers who occupied this area have been found to exhibit high levels of bone infections (Anderson & Borns, 1997).

Borrelia gets into bones and joints by twisting in like a corkscrew. Researchers (Marre et al, 2010) have looked into the role of inflammation caused by *Borrelia* and found that adrenomedullin, a protein produced in response to infection, plays an active role in antimicrobial activity and in the regulation of inflammatory processes. Patients with untreated Lyme arthritis have been found to have a higher level of adrenomedullin in their synovial fluid, which causes a marked swelling in infected joints. Adrenomedullin may help *Borrelia* to avoid immune system attacks. This effect on the immune system's inflammatory processes may be involved in the development of chronic Lyme arthritis in some patients. Other processes implicated in Lyme disease, osteoarthritis, rheumatoid arthritis, gout, and ankylosing spondylitis, include the effects of Toll Like Receptors (TLRs) to drive pro-inflammatory cytokine production in infected or injured tissues (McCormack, et al, 2009).

Blood serum reactivity against the Outer Surface Protein A [OspA] antigen of a *Borrelia* infection is associated with the pathogenesis of rheumatoid arthritis [RA]. Chronic Lyme arthritis may be a result of an antibody to OspA cross-reacting with the synovial tissue found in many large human joints. In synovial joints, bones are enclosed in a fibrous capsule that is filled with fluid that cushions the bones' articulating surfaces. These joints seem to be especially vulnerable for attack. This may be because antibodies cross-react with OspA antigen, creating an auto-immune reaction. The blood of patients with RA is more likely to contain Immunoglobulin G that was reactive against OspA antigens than that of patients with other autoimmune diseases. Various studies have shown that people who experience Lyme arthritis develop an OspA specific antibody that correlates directly with the severity and duration of the arthritis. Although joint inflammation in patients with Lyme disease and RA might result from the effect of the OspA antibody, the arthritic damage might also be due to the antibodies being directed against joint antigens. One such antigen is cytokeratin 10 (Hsieh, 2007). It has been found that cytokeratin 10, cross reacts with OspA (Ghosh, 2006).

Because of this, Lyme patients may develop systemic autoimmune joint diseases like rheumatoid arthritis, psoriatic

arthritis, and peripheral spondyloarthritis (Arvikar, 2016). Even dogs with clinical signs of polyarthritis sometimes develop rheumatoid arthritis subsequent to *Borrelia* infection (Rouch, 1989).

Lyme infection directly affects bones by decreasing bone formation, lowering bone density and stunted bone formation. The mechanism through which *Borrelia* decreases bone has been studied using a murine[mouse] model. Researchers tested the bones of mice infected with *Borrelia* for bacterial DNA. They analyzed the dense bones characterized by a thin shaft that in humans make up the legs and arms, as well as vertebra. The study found the same levels of *Borrelia* DNA in the bones as previous studies had found in other body tissues like the skin. Bone mass density measurements were significantly correlated with the amount of *Borrelia* DNA harbored in bones. *Borrelia* bacterial colonization of bone was correlated with loss of bone mass, contributing to bone porosity. *Borrelia* were found to inhibit or mutate the production of osteoblasts, which are specialized cells that make more bone, while allowing osteoclasts, the specialized cells that breaks down bone, to remain normal. Bone loss may result from less bone-building by osteoblasts. In this model, osteoclast activity would continue in infected bones, but the degraded osteoids (subunits of bone architecture) would not be replaced at the normal rate because not enough osteoblasts would be working to reform the bone (Tang, et al, 2017).

Borrelia also attacks collagen. The proteoglycan aggrecan forms a major component of cartilage and plays a key role in protecting collagen from degradation (Pratta et al, 2003b). Aggrecan forms large aggregated complexes which fill the collagen meshwork of the body. The aggrecan molecule contains multiple glycosaminoglycan (GAG) side chains, which allow it to swell against the type II collagen scaffold in the presence of water. This is what gives articular cartilage the ability to resist compressive forces during joint loading (Roughley, 2001). Aggrecan degradation is one of the key events underlying the pathogenesis of Lyme arthritis (Bondeson et al, 2008; Caterson et al, 2000; Sandy, 2003).

Lyme disease spirochetes possess aggrecan-binding proteins. Two *Borrelial* binding proteins: the Extracellular Matrix Ligand Bgp (BB0588) and a protease BbHtrA (BB0104) that is expressed during infection is conserved in the three major Lyme disease spirochete species. BbHtrA cleaves aggrecan and destroys its function (Russell & Johnson, 2013). The spirochetes activate metalloproteases, which cause collagen to dissolve and then colonize it in micro-colonies within collagen fibers. They inhibit the regeneration of collagen and delay the healing process or prevent it completely. Bone marrow is made of a collagen matrix. *Borrelia* infection is implicated in skeletal remains by the appearance of scar damage on the bones of untreated infected animals, especially in the joint areas. Severe Lyme infection causes bone loss, porosity, and lesions. The host inflammatory response seen in Lyme arthritis has an acute clinical presentation similar to that of other septic arthritis, especially in children. The knee is the most commonly affected joint, with involvement in up to ninety percent of patients. The elbow, ankle, hip, and wrist may also be affected (Willis, A.A. et al, 2003).

In historic skeletal remains, autoimmune Lyme arthritis and rheumatoid arthritis may be indistinguishable from each other (Chary-Valckenaere, 1997) but there is a lot of evidence for bone infection. While the hallmark of osteoarthritis [OA] is a condition known as eburnation- a smooth area caused by two bones coming into contact and rubbing against each other, it also occurs in Rheumatoid Arthritis [RA] and Lyme Arthritis [LA]. The hallmark of Lyme/rheumatoid arthritis is bone damage from inflammation and/or infection accompanied by eburnation. On the femoral bone head, eburnated surface is actually less extensive in OA than in RA or LA at an advanced stage. Osteophytes [bone spurs] can occur in all there types of arthritis due to disregulation of bone growth (Lagier, 2006).

LA peripheral poly-arthritis lesions (scars from infectious damage to the ends of multiple bones) have been found on a set of human skeletal remains from Alabama that date to 5,000 B.C. (Rothschild, et al. 1988). Another possible diagnosis of Lyme disease as the cause of similar pathological bone conditions, comes

from a later prehistoric Tchefuncte Indian adolescent skeleton found in Louisiana. It dates from between 500 and 300 A.D (Lewis, B, 1994). There is such a large cluster of pre-contact skeletons with infected joints in southwestern Kentucky, West-central Tennessee, and Northwestern Alabama from the Archaic period (5000-500 BC), with a minor spread to Ohio in the Woodland period (500 BC-AD 1000), followed by an explosive spread after the late 18th century, that that area has been labeled 'The Cradle of Rheumatoid Arthritis (Rothschild, 1991). It could just as easily be called the "Cradle of Lyme Disease" for North America.

As the glaciers melted after the last Ice Age, tick-risky habitat moved northward on the continent and this geographic area came to be covered by a deciduous forest as the climate warmed. Various Native American groups from this geographical area have folkloric stories that define a clear link of deer with arthritic conditions. In a traditional Creek story, hunters are warned to be cautious with deer because they have mysterious powers. If a hunter does not show proper respect when he has killed a deer, it would cause him rheumatism and the hunter would be forced to walk the rest of his life with aches and pains. Another Native group, the Cherokee, once occupied parts of Appalachia. Cherokee folklore contains both the strong admonition against touching the skin of a diseased deer and the following story about respecting the spirit of slain deer:

Little Deer, the chief of the deer and the animal spirit who took vengeance on unthinking hunters, ran as swiftly as the wind to a deer just killed. Bending over the blood spots on the ground, Little Deer asked the spirit of the deer if it had heard the hunter make amends, the proper prayer. If the answer was yes, then Little Deer left. If no, Little Deer followed the trail of blood left by the hunter who then carried the deer to the hunter's door, where he "[put] into the hunters body the spirit of rheumatism that shall rack him with aches and pains from that time henceforth"(Ketch, 2000).

There are litanies of Native American herbal treatments for arthritis and rheumatism showing that these were diseases that indigenous people confronted and treated. Some of these Native cures, like bearberry and goldenseal, have mildly antibiotic properties that would possibly be somewhat effective for treating

Lyme disease (Weiner & Weiner, 1994). Examination of historical medical texts and descriptions of practices that were found in Europe, the Central Asian Steppes, and in China show a linkage between arthritis symptoms and "cures" that have antibiotic properties.

In Europe, it appears that the Greeks and Romans, living in southern, highly modified, and urban landscapes that produced the founding fathers of Western Medicine had little arthritis or rheumatism. The only rheumatic disease clearly identified by Hippocrates is gout. Of the 412 Aphorisms, only six refer to anything resembling Lyme or rheumatism-like disorders:

-In the elderly: dyspnoea, catarrh and coughing, dysuria, joint pain, kidney inflammation, vertigo, etc.

-Swelling and joint pain, ulcers, those of a gouty nature and muscle strain are usually improved by cold water, which reduces swelling and eliminates the pain, as a moderate degree of numbness eliminates pain.

-In gouty disorders, inflammation disappears within 40 days.

-Typically, gouty disorders are exacerbated in the spring and autumn.(Hippocrates, 470 - 410 B.C.).

Another Greek physician, Dioscorides, who worked in Rome during the 1st century AD was the author of the book *De Materia Medica,* a treatise that might be considered the source of western herbal medicine knowledge. He recommended using ivy against what seems to be osteoarthritis of the hips. Ground Ivy is an effective antimicrobial and anti-inflammatory. European physicians recommended, from the time of Hippocrates on, willow bark to treat fever and pain, perhaps including rheumatic or osteoarthritic pain. This treatment was used by the Neanderthals and has found its way into the Era of Scientific Medicine as aspirin.

Some preserved skeletons dating from the Pharaonic era in Egypt show that ankylosing spondylitis, an inflammatory disease affecting the joints of the lumbar region that had afflicted the

Neanderthal still existed in the third millennium BC. Egyptian documents reveal that joint pain was treated with ointments containing fat, oil, honey or bone marrow. Honey is an effective antimicrobial (Mandal & Mandal, 2011).

Arthritis seems to have became a rare occurrence in the orderly organized landscapes of Middle Age Europe, even amongst hard working peasant laborers. A study of the skeletons of two hundred and fifty two individuals who lived in the town of Bernau in Brandenburg (now Germany) from between the 13th and 16th centuries, show that their main activities were agriculture and crafts, which provided them with relatively good living conditions for their time. But life expectancy, in the age of the Black Death, was low. Fifty two percent of the individuals studied had died before the age of twenty years and life expectancy was only twenty five years (Faber, et al. 2003).

A study of two hundred and seventy three adult skeletons that lived between the Neolithic [onset of agrarian lifestyle] and the Middle Ages also shows the absence of arthritis in large joints and an absence of rheumatoid arthritis and ankylosing spondylitis (Kramer,et al.1990). In a much larger series of skeletons [six hundred and ninety five Saxon or of the English Middle Ages], British researchers found signs of osteoarthritis of the hip in only twenty nine of them. Knee arthritis was present in only four cases. The authors of that study concluded that arthritis of the knee may actually be of recent onset (Rogers & Dieppe,September 1994).

William of Baillou (1538-1616), Dean of the Faculty of Medicine of Paris, used the word "rheumatism" in the modern sense for the first time in western medicine. In his book, *Liber de rheumatismo et pleuritide dorsali,* he designates acute rheumatoid arthritis but his description shows that it was attached to the old Hippocratic theory of the humors:

The humors (especially blood) flowing through the body provoke severe pain with their harmful substances. The condition we wrongly call catarrh should be called rheumatism. Rheumatism is a kind of disease of fluid receptacles in which the malignant humors flowing from inside to outside the body are deposited in the extremities and joints. What gout represents for a particular extremity, rheumatism represents for the entire body.

Those malignant humors included *Borrelia* spirochetes. Recently, it has been found that spirochetes can be detected in ancient bones if you look for it using stain, direct light microscope, and dark field illumination, even when DNA is unlikely to survive. Spirochetes have been found associated with a seven thousand year old European skeleton (Gaul,et al. 2011).

Another study traced long-term trends in arthritis in North America using a large set of skeletal samples spanning from prehistoric times to the present. Knee arthritis existed at low frequencies, but since the Mid-Twentieth Century, the disease has doubled in prevalence. While the recent surge in knee osteoarthritis has been hypothesized to have occurred simply because people live longer and are more commonly obese, it may be more complex. This study concluded that additional risk factors that have become ubiquitous within the last half-century need to be studied further. Increases in longevity and BMI are insufficient to explain the approximate doubling of knee osteoarthritis prevalence. Prevention will require research on additional independent risk factors that either arose or have become amplified in the Postindustrial Era. This should include automobile usage and Lyme disease as variables (Wallace, et al., 2017).

The trend in arthritis throughout history seems to be related to interactions with ticks:

Somewhat High for Hunter-gathers,

Diminished AFTER the Agrarian Revolution,

Low during the managed landscape of the Middle Ages,

High after The Black Death,

Almost non-existent during Industrialization, but has

Skyrocketed since the middle of the Twentieth Century.

This may be directly related to human interactions with peri-domestic tick-risky landscapes.

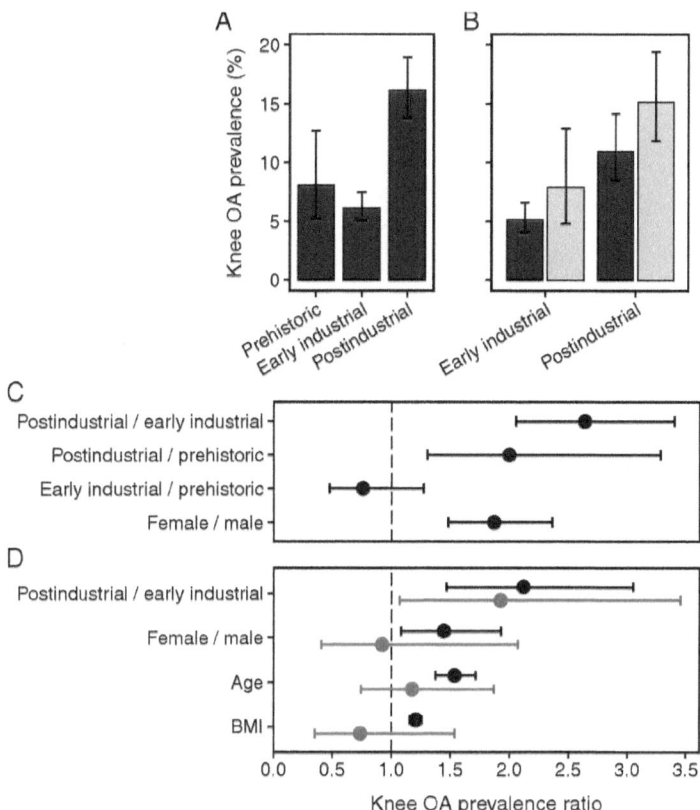

Figure 31. Knee-arthritis prevalence during different time periods. (*A* and *B*) Prevalence from regression models controlling for sex (*A*) as well as age, BMI, sex, and ethnicity (*B*). Dark and light gray bars are from unmatched and matched analyses, respectively (*B*).(*C* and *D*) Prevalence ratios from regression models including sex (*C*) as well as age, BMI[weight], sex, and ethnicity (*D*) as predictor variables. Black and light gray dots are from unmatched and matched analyses, respectively (*D*). Age and BMI were entered into models as continuous variables, but effects are reported for 10-y and 5-U intervals, respectively (*D*). Whiskers represent 95% Confidence Intervals. (Wallace, et al, 2017).

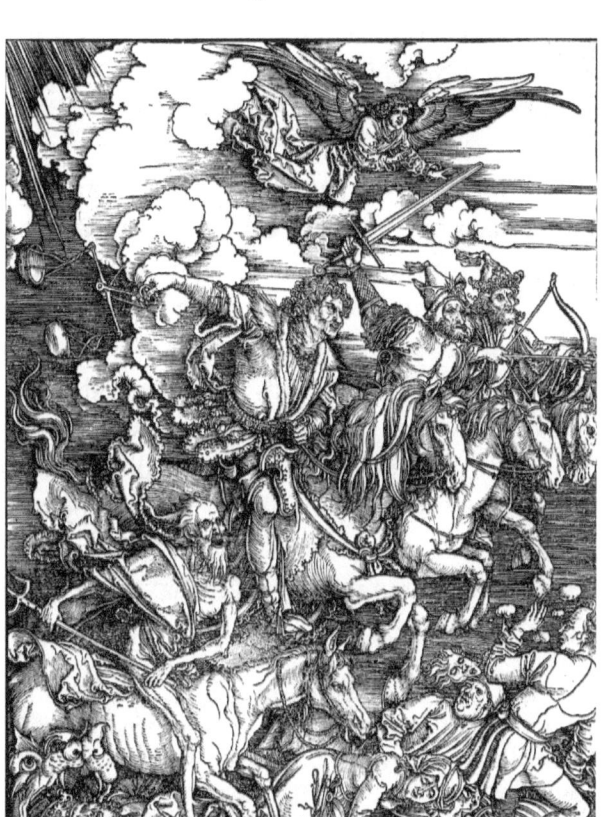

Figure 32. *The Four Horsemen of the Apocalypse.* Albrecht Durer, circa 1497–98. "They were given power over a fourth of the earth to kill by sword, famine, plague, and by the wild beasts of the earth." Revelations 6: 7-8.

CHILDREN OF THE GRASS

In the Bible, the end of the world is envisioned as arriving on horseback. Revelations Chapter 6, Verses 7 and 8 describe a set of four horsemen who sweep in bringing war, starvation, pestilence and the spread of wild beasts. These horsemen may be a cultural memory of events that occurred thousands of years before the

Bible was written, when Yamnaya horsemen from the grassy steppes of Central Asia swept both the East and the West, creating an apocalypse for those standing in their path. They brought with them archery skills, metalworking technologies [they probably cast some of the first bronze swords] and an expansive trading network leading all the way across Eurasia to China. The bow, sword, and weighing scales that three horsemen carry represent those three cultural activities. They would bring about an almost complete male genetic transformation in some geographic areas, as well as a culinary shift-away from grain towards the increased consumption of dairy and meat. They brought with them herds of cattle, sheep, and horses that must have outcompeted local wild deer for space.

The Yamnaya brought death in the form of virulent diseases, especially smallpox and pneumonic plague, which they may have had some immunity from, but which reeked havoc on naive populations. This is described dramatically by an early filmmaker:

The horseman on the white horse was clad in a showy and barbarous attire. While his horse continued galloping, he was bending his bow in order to spread pestilence abroad. At his back swung the brass quiver filled with poisoned arrows, containing the germs of all diseases (Ibáñez, 1916).

The Yamnaya most likely had little experience with Lyme disease before they arrived in Northern Europe. *Ixodes* ticks and the *Borrelia* that they carry thrive in deciduous forests and eschew grasslands. Species that evolve within good tick habitat (Lane & Quistad, February, 1998) seem to have immune systems that have co-evolved with various tick-borne infections. Others do not.

The modern human's immune system is the product of genetic and cultural fusions that have occurred over millennia. The horsemen that swept into Europe may be partially responsible for some of our immune system's trouble handling *Borrelia*. For eons, the Yamnaya immune system had encountered plague and poxes but very few *Ixodes* ticks because of their grass based lifestyle, the use of fire, and protective clothing choices. They brought their own pathogens with them when they arrived in Europe seven thousand

years ago, being preceded by a pandemic that killed off a large part of the European Agrarian population and resulted in an almost complete turnover of Y haplotypes in many areas of Northern Europe. In return, they got exposed to Lyme Disease.

There is much debate about whether or not the grasslands of the earth were the cradle of humanity. Since the discovery of some seven million year old fossilized teeth and the jaw of a new potential hominid called *Graecopithecus* that lived its life north of the Mediterranean Sea (Fuss J, et al., 2017), along with some 9.7 million year old teeth in Germany (Embury-Dennis, October 19, 2017), it seems that hominids developed over a larger and more varied geographical landscape than had previously been hypothesized.

But the emergence of early humans does seem to coincide with the expansion of grassy savannas and steppes- dry grasslands mixed with trees- across both East Africa and in Eastern Europe. Researchers have speculated that these grasslands may hold the key to human evolution. The expansion of savannas may have forced our ancestors to begin walking upright to see over the grass, which in turn, freed up their hands for creative tool use. *Graecopithecus* ate dry and hard grassland vegetation and developed teeth with wide molars and thick enamel that are unlike those of other great apes that evolved eating softer forest grown foods (Anglin, 2017).

The story of our more recent grass based ancestry begins when Early Modern Humans arrived in Central Asia. It may have been at about 70,000 years BP, when Mt. Toba in Indonesia, erupted and spewed a thick layer of dust into the earth's atmosphere where it blocked sunlight. This caused death and a human genetic bottleneck (Ambrose, Stanley H., 1998). A thousand year abrupt cooling event, a massive drought or some unknown epidemic may have driven people out of Africa. Most scientists agree that, whatever the cause, by approximately 65,000 years ago, Early Modern Humans began to make a series of migrations out of Africa, with some groups interacting with the Neanderthals and Denisovans in Central Asia. (Rogers, et al, 2017).

They were hunter-gatherers who may have followed herds of grass eating animals. Human migration in the northern hemisphere was influenced by a series of re-occurring glaciation events. The final one is called the Last Glacial Maxima. During this time, humans survived in areas called refuges. One was an ice free area of grassland that is in modern day Ukraine, Russia, and Uzbekistan. There, in isolation, they developed a unique culture and enough Single Nucleotide Polymorphisms built up for their district Y haplotypes to evolve.

DNA haplotypes can be useful tools for tracing the migrations of people as well as various animals over time. Haplotypes develop among groups of animals that live in specific geographic areas for long periods of time. Small shared mutations, called Single Nucleotide Polymorphisms [SNP]accumulate over time. Humans clock in at about two per generation.

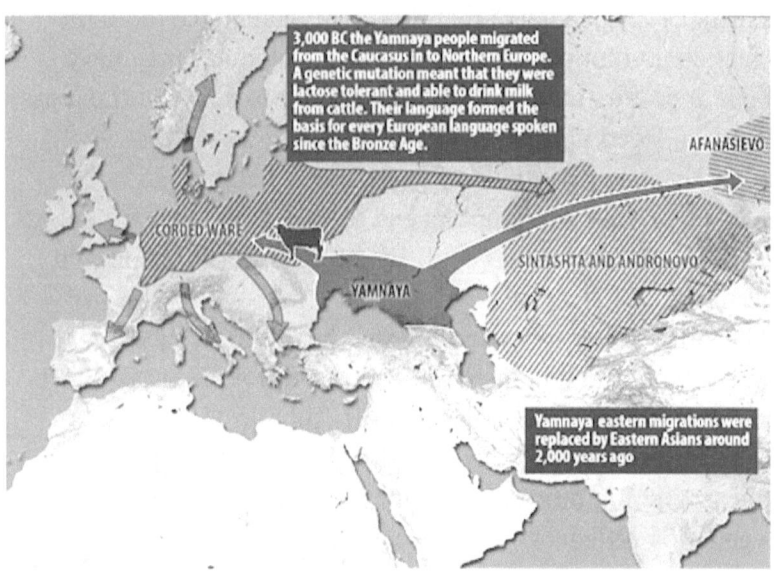

Figure 33. The Great Yamnaya Migrations. www.geneticgeneology.com

When enough SNP's add up to create a big enough difference, a distinct haplotype is formed. Scientists have been about to trace the movement of horses, cattle, chickens and humans over time by examining prevailing DNA haplotypes.

The domestication of cattle and horses, part of the "Neolithic Revolution," started about 11000 years ago. DNA has been used to trace the animals that were domesticated. For example, the now extinct wild auroch, *Bos primigenius* (the last specimen was shot in 1627 AD in Poland) was the ancestor of all domesticated cows. *Bos indices* is the the humped-back cow of Asia and Africa. The Taurine breeds, *Bos taurus* (Taurus is a mountain range in southern Turkey), are the ancestors of the modern dairy cow. The highest genetic variability among cattle is found in the Near East, which identifies it as the likely origin for European cattle (Troy et al., 2001).

Cattle were domesticated at 10,000 BP and sheep/goats at 11,000 BP. Scientists have located the origin of domesticated sheep in the upper Euphrates Valley of south-eastern Turkey. Geneticists have retraced the path of migration routes for domesticated cattle from Turkey into theBalkans, then along a northern line following the Danube River and a southern line following the Adriatic coast (Zeder,2008).

Human populations have varied evolutionary histories and, more importantly, have co-evolved with different combinations of animals and microbes. Hence, the repertoire of genetic alleles and epigenetic switches that afford resistance or susceptibility to pathogens will vary in different populations depending upon their evolutionary history (Trueba, G., 2014).

This brings us to the haplotypes of the last great horse ridden migration into Western Asia and Europe-which went almost unrecognized before the advent of modern genetic research. One puzzling result of advances in DNA research has been the finding that, when analyzing the graves of members of earlier settlements, the genomes they were finding did not share many similarities with the modern-day populations that occupied the same geographical location, especially within the male Y haplotypes. This led to the

realization that there had been a near total population change in Europe that occurred beginning in around 5000 BP. The large demographic change happened as a result of massive migrations of people from the Pontiac-Caspian steppes into Neolithic Europe. Importantly, it may have been preceded by an unrecorded, particularly deadly, and widespread unknown epidemic of unknown origin: an early horse ridden apocalypse.

After hundreds of thousands of years of pre-historic human cultural growth in Europe, DNA research and a fresh look at recorded history has found the turn over. The majority of modern Europeans owe their ancestry to a group of Pot Smoking Dispersed living Individualistic Bronze Age Cowboys- The Yamnaya. Here the R male Y haplotype and a very distinct culture developed: they were a set of great nomadic horse breeding and cattle and sheep herding people. When they swept west out of the Eurasian grasslands into Europe, they may have been brought an unknown epidemic. It may have been a simmering form of pneumonic plague that had been passed person to person along trading contacts and routes that stretched all the way back through Central Asia to China. They could also have carried some virulent pox viruses. They may have acquired "herd" immunity because of childhood cases of cowpox.

Change is a complex process. Warfare may have been involved. Evidence for a major, and previously unknown, large scale Bronze Age battle in the Tollense Valley of Germany dating back to 1250 BC, has recently been found (Gannon, 2017, October 23). However it happened, young Yamnaya men seem to have become attached with young agriculturalist women. Their offspring went on to found many of the later well known cultures of Europe- Cordware and Bell Beaker. These Yamnaya were recently found hiding in plain sight. It just took a bit of genetic detective work to find them.

A study published in 2015 found that the DNA from one hundred and one Bronze Age skeletons showed that Europeans, especially Northern Europeans, descended genetically from the horse loving nomadic tribes. Studies of Yamnaya genetics have found that the paternal haplotype lineages that begin with R1b and

R1a, as well as Indo-European languages, and metal working technologies were brought into Europe during the Bronze Age. DNA studies found that they contributed seventy three percent of the ancestral contribution of DNA to Corded Ware skeletal remains found in Germany. The same study estimated a forty to fifty four percent ancestral contribution of Yamnaya DNA to modern Central & Northern Europeans, and a twenty to thirty two percent contribution to modern Southern Europeans. Only the Sardinians measure at less than ten percent. In Europe, they are the cultural and genetic ancestors of both the Celts and the Scythians, who in turn, are considered the Fathers of the Anglo Saxons (Gibbons, 2017). The Yamnaya also contributed to groups that migrated east, with an estimated thirty to fifty percent steppe related admixture found among modern Northern South Asians and between six and twenty percent in modern Southern Asians (Allentoft, et al., 2015). There is even a small group of R Y haplotype Africans.they did however, seem to carry fewer Neanderthal immunity genes than some other groups.

  This genetic 'takeover' of Northern Europe by the R Y-haplotypes may relate to modern Lyme disease incidence.Archaic-like alleles underlie differences in the expression of TLR genes and are associated with increased microbial resistance in large cohorts. This provides strong evidence for recurrent adaptive introgression at the TLR1, 6, 10 locus, resulting in differences in disease phenotypes between modern human groups. In Europe, a North-South gradient is apparent with significantly population differentiation between Southern Europeans and all other European groups. Finnish and British have frequencies between 14.8% and 26.4% while Iberians are at over thirty nine percent . The frequency of Archaic haplotypes is higher in the Southern European populations that also have less Yamnaya ancestry. In Asia, the more Eastern populations (Japanese and Han Chinese, frequency 53.4% and 53.6%) show high differentiation from other Asian populations (frequency 21.7%–41.9%).

  The variation introduced by introgression from Archaic Humans might have been an important factor in the adaptation of modern humans to novel pathogens in challenging new

environments. Introgressed alleles seems to enhance innate immune surveillance and reactivity against certain pathogens, but that this might also have increased hypersensitivity to non-pathogenic allergens, resulting in some allergic diseases in present-day people (Danneman, et al 2016). The Yamnaya migration may have created a mismatch between immunity and prevailing pathogens that is still evident, especially when confronting *Borrelia* and other tick-borne infections..

The movement of some wild animal haplotypes can also be linked to this Yamnaya migration. Migrating humans do not move alone. They bring along a full panoply of bacteria and a set of other species, both intentionally and unintentionally. An example is the striped field mouse (Apodemus agrarius), which colonized northwestern Europe beginning in around 6500 BP. This mouse has become common on the southern Danish Islands of Lolland and Falster, where they were isolated from mainland Europe. When a set of full mitochondrial genomes were sequenced from these mice, phylogenetic relationships and estimated divergence time supported human-induced colonization from the Steppes to Denmark during the Subatlantic or Subboreal period. This was the time of the large Yamnaya migrations (Andersen, 2017).

Although today's Google Earth satellite view shows that the Eurasian steppe is a vast expanse of desert and mostly rectangular shaped fields that have been created by centuries of human actions- five thousand years ago it was a vast treeless swath of varied grasslands that extended from the mouth of the Danube River in Europe across to Mongolia. When they became agriculturalists, it was as a nomadic herding people tied to their herds, not their land or crops. Wool processing and horseback riding were in practice on the Steppes by the Bronze Age. They were metal workers. Copper deposits were mined and the ore was processed into a variety of tools and artifacts.These innovations created a broadly similar culture from Eastern Europe to the borders of China. The people who inhabited the part of this geographic area located directly above the Black Sea, are called Kurgan [Russian word for the burial mound (barrow) covering a pit grave], or Yamnaya, which

simply means "mound burial." They developed a cultural practice of burying their dead in pits that were then covered over by

distinctive mounds that were placed along important herding routes.

The Yamnaya were true children of the grasslands. They occupied their landscape with an individualistic, pastoral, dispersed, scattered and mobile pattern that was based upon small groups of nuclear families and their herds of cattle, sheep, and especially, horses. This culture was already formed when the European climate was transitioning from a warmer/ wetter weather pattern to a consistently drier/colder period. Climatologists call this the Atlantic/Subboreal transition and date it as occurring in about 3000 BC. The Yamnaya moved around in search of better pasturage for their animals, which led them into Europe. Herds were dispersed over large areas, which meant that large herds could be owned and wealth could be on the hoof, not by owning land or stationary property.This mobile residency pattern and movement away from river valleys was facilitated by the wheel, wagons, felt tents, and woolen clothing (Anthony, 2007).

Wagons were a critically important innovation, because they permitted a herder to carry enough food, shelter, and water to remain with his herd. Wool clothing made it easier to live in the open steppe and horseback riding was facilitated by the innovation of trousers. Innovations in metallurgy created technological advantages for this group of people and they participated in a thriving trade network that later became the Silk Road leading across to China, that was centered upon trade in cannabis, which they may have gathered while moving through their landscape (Dilworth, 2010). It may have helped them to stay healthy.

While research examining the effect of cannabis on the specific *Borrelia* bacteria that causes Lyme disease is lacking, cannabinoids have shown efficacy against many types of bacteria. One study found that both tetrahydro cannabinol (THC) and cannabidiol (CBD) strongly reduce the activity of streptococci. Another study found cannabis to have antibacterial effects against *Bacillus subtilis, Pseudomonas aeruginosa,* and *Aspergillus niger.*

Most recently, a study found cannabis extract to exert

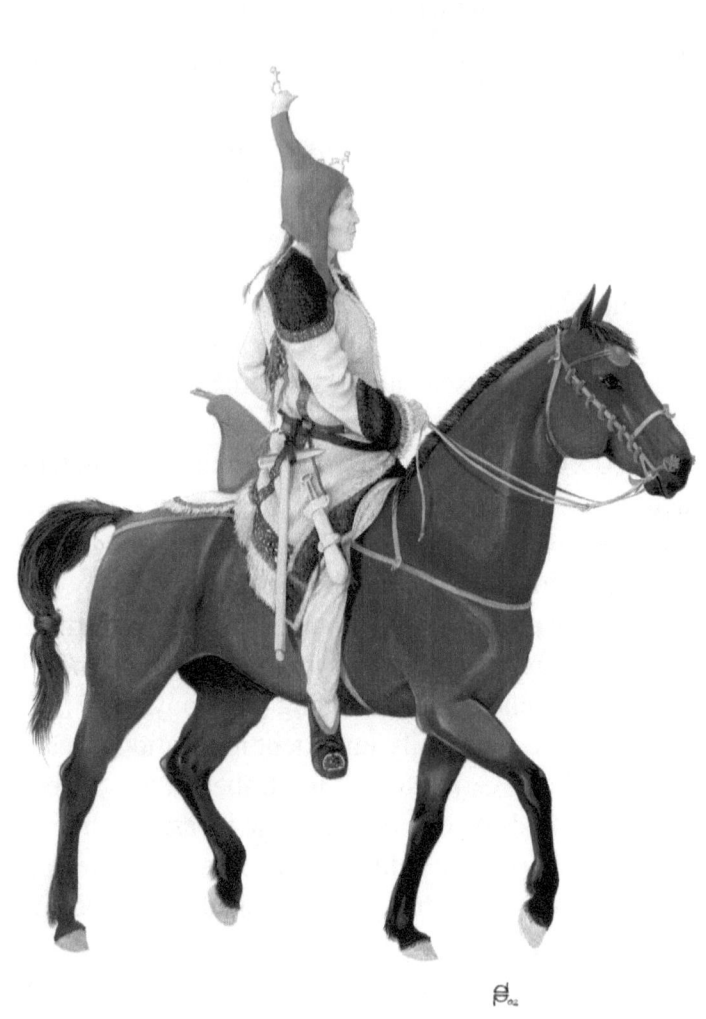

Figure 34. The Yamnaya were the ancestors of the Scythians, who in turn, were the ancestors of the Anglo-Saxons. A Scythian rider wore clothing that left them well protected from ticks. Courtesy British Museum, 2017.

pronounced antibacterial activity against *Staphylococcus aureus, Pseudomonas aeruginosa, Escherichia coli*, and *Enterococcus faecalis*(Ali, E.M, et al., 2012). Cannabis usage was continued on the Steppes over time and seems to have been used medicinally. Two of the Kurgen mummies from around 2000 years ago displayed signs of cancer. One woman was buried with a brazier containing charred hemp [cannabis?] suggesting they recognized the pain killing effect of the smoke.

Analysis of other human remains from excavated kurgan graves show that they suffered from toothaches and bovine tuberculosis. They may have used koumiss –a cultured milk product similar to Kefir, that remained the most effective treatment for tuberculosis in Russia before antibiotics were discovered (Schlott, et al., 2007).

Population genomics offer insights on Yamnaya physical and physiological traits. The ability to digest milk[lactose tolerance] into adulthood is nearly universal among Northern Europeans today. Before the Yamnaya migration, it was rare in Europeans, contradicting earlier claims that the trait helped early European farmers to gain calories from milk. Of the one hundred and one sequenced Bronze Age individuals, the Yamnaya were most likely to have the DNA variation responsible for lactose tolerance, hinting that the steppe migrants might have introduced that trait into Europe (Gibbons, 2015).

When the Yamnaya headed east, the upheaval that followed their arrival in Central Asia may have even exceeded the transformation that followed the European colonization of the Americas. Changes in Central Asia during the early and middle Bronze Age were "extremely abrupt," which could be due to war,disease or climate change but was definitely associated with the arrival of The Yamnaya." Central Asians were hunter-gatherers using stone tools and the Yamnaya suddenly came in with horses, wagons, wheels and bronze weapons (Allentoft, et al, 2015).

The Yamnaya's effects were less striking in Northern Europe,which was already populated by farmers, but they did change the way people buried their dead, added pottery styles,

changed the material they used for creating tools and weapons, changed the type of housing they lived in, settlement patterns, and family structure. They turned the horse into an important folkloric icon that made its way into mythology, the Bible, was carved into the hillsides of England, and has survived to the modern day (Kristiansen, et al. 2017). Before the introduction of the automobile, a conquering military hero was most often depicted on horseback. The Yamnaya often buried humans with horse remains. Until recently, the remains of the Yamnaya had been assigned to the world of archaeology.

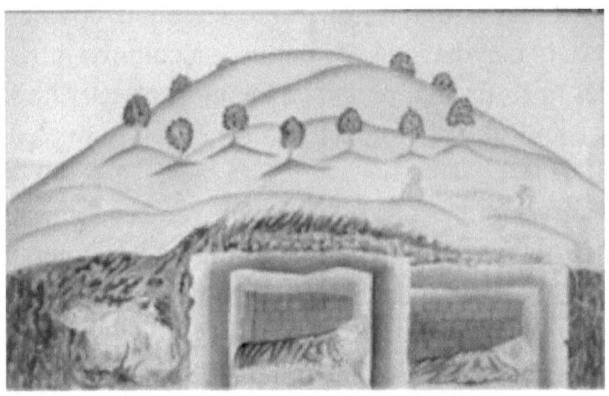

Figure 35. Artist's impression of a burial mound. In Ukraine they are called Kurgen, in England, Barrows. Watercolor illustration, 18th century. Russian Academy of Sciences.

Some of their pit graves have been excavated. Human burials seem to have been accompanied by ritual feasting-graves included animal bones from sheep, cattle and horses. A pipe with the remnants of burned cannabis have been found in one grave along with cords made from hemp. Seeds of wheat and millet have been found in the clay of some Pit Grave pots which may represent grain collection and/or that some early agriculture was being practiced in the steppe river valleys.

As the climate changed and resource scarcity created pressure from more Eastern steppe tribes, the Yamnaya began a mass migration west into Northern Europe taking their cattle, horses, and even steppe mice with them. As they moved in, they burned forests to create grazing lands, killing off *Ixodes* ticks they

might have been harboring. By about 2000 BC, they began to settle in place with a scattered dispersed pattern. The Yamnaya faded into history, remembered partially as the Scythian Culture which is a fusion of Yamnaya with a group called the Sintashta, and as influencing the Celtic and Cordedware cultures of Northern Europe. The Sintashta were the innovators of the use of the horse drawn chariot in warfare-a technology which spread throughout Europe and Asia. The red haired Tocharian mummies found in the Tarim Basin burials in China may have been part of the Sintashta cultural group (Anthony, 2009).

The Yamnaya migration occurred at a time of climatic decline. In 3200 BC, temperatures on Earth plunged. In fact, they plunged so fast that it flash-froze plants which scientist later found in perfectly preserved condition. It was at about this time that Otzi's dead body was flash-frozen and thus he was influenced by the same event. Whatever happened to the climate, it was abrupt and very large-scale. Ice cores taken from Tanzania's Mount Kilimanjaro ice fields show that another catastrophic drought devastated the tropics. This may have been linked to a volcanic eruption of the Avachinsky, Kamchatka, Russia volcano. Scientists have found a huge spike in sulfate concentration in dust captured in Greenland ice from that time. One of the initial explosive eruptions produced a layer of basaltic andesite tephra which was dispersed at a distance of more than 300 km to the north and formed one of the main marker tephra layers for this area (Bazanova LI, et al., 2004).

In an oak tree ring chronology from Ireland, an index of tree ring narrowness peaks at about 3150 BC, again suggesting a major climatic event at this time. An arid interval 5010-4860 (+/- 150) is found at Tigalmamine in Morocco. Corresponding decline of oaks (*Quercus*) in favor of grasses (*Gramineae*) suggests reduced winter precipitation corresponding to cooler sea temperatures in the North Atlantic (Lamb, H. F. et al, 1995). Farming collapse due to climatic change may have led to famine, human and animal immuno-impairment, and may have been followed by Yamnaya introduced plague.

Migrants from far away places bring viruses and bacteria

with them that can have a big impact on a local population who have not developed the same kind of resistance to infection. If pneumonic plague was carried along as part of the Yamnaya migrations, it would have had devastating effects on the groups that they encountered. Well-documented cases have shown the pneumonic plague's chain of infection can go from a single hunter or herder to ravaging an entire community in just two to three days (Rasmussen et al., October 22, 2015).

Archaeologists have found that an early form of the bacteria *Yersinia pestis* may have been passed from person to person and spread from western China to the steppes (Valtuena et al., December, 2016).The first indication of plague anywhere in Europe is found in the Baltic region and coincides with the time of the arrival of the steppe population component (Allentoft et al., 2015). Two late Neolithic *Yersinia pestis* genomes in this study were reconstructed from individuals associated with the Corded Ware Complex (Gyvakarai1 and KunilaII). The Baltic genomes are genetically derived from a strain that came from the Altai region, suggesting that the disease spread with steppe pastoralists from Central Eurasia to Eastern and Central Europe during their massive range expansion.The younger Late Neolithic *Yersinia pestis* genomes found in Southern Germany are genetically derived from the Baltic strains and are found in individuals associated with the later Bell Beaker Complex (Allentoft et al., 2015; Haak et al., 2015). The youngest of all the plague genomes (RISE505), found also in the Altai region, descends from Central European strains suggesting a later spread back into the eastern steppes, probably along trade routes.

This plague of five thousand years ago, combined with the climatic downturn, created what must have seemed like an apocalypse. The Yamnaya, who may have acquired some degree of immunity and who lived in a dispersed pattern that was less amenable to person to person infection, were not as affected. At the point when *Yersinia pestis* mutated into a flea borne pathogen spread on the back of rats, the Yamnaya would also have also been somewhat protected by their horsey lifestyle. They, especially the men, lived in close proximity to their horses which may have

made them less hospitable to plague carrying fleas. Fleas avoid horses. The Yamnaya also probably smelled of horse much of the time-a natural flea repellent.

Equus ferus, the extinct wild ancestor of domestic horses, was born in East Asia. The original founder population of the domestic horse was established in the western Eurasian Steppe and mixed with local wild stocks as they spread throughout Europe and Asia. Herds were repeatedly restocked with wild horses. Horse domestication became widespread in a short period of time and the expansion of the domestic horse and horse related technology throughout Europe was little short of explosive. In the space of about 500 years, for example, there is evidence that horse-drawn chariot technology spread from the steppes to Greece, Egypt, and Mesopotamia. By another 500 years, the horse-drawn chariot had spread across to China (Achilli, et al., 2012).

As a culture and genome that developed in a drier grassland environment, the Yamnaya would have had encountered few tick-borne infections in their lifetimes. There were simply fewer ticks about in the grassy steppes and fewer acceptable blood meal hosts necessary for tick survival. For unknown reasons, *Ixodes* ticks even give steppe mice a wide berth when it comes to blood meal attachment (Egyed, 2017).

Ixodid ticks and the *Borrelia* that they carry evolved within specific environmental areas. Species that also evolved within these areas, like the white tailed deer, white footed mouse, or even western fence lizards (Lane and Quistad, February, 1998) have immune system that have co-evolved with various tick-borne infections. Some human haplotypes, like those represented in the Yamnaya, evolved outside risky areas and produce immune systems that may be naive when it comes to dealing with tick-borne infections. Others have immune systems that can over-react and end up with autoimmune dysfunction. Either way, many humans, as children of the grass find *Borrelia* to be a daunting opponent. The use of cannabis as medicine has deep deep roots that began on the steppes of Central Asia and were transplanted into western culture by the pioneering Yamnaya.

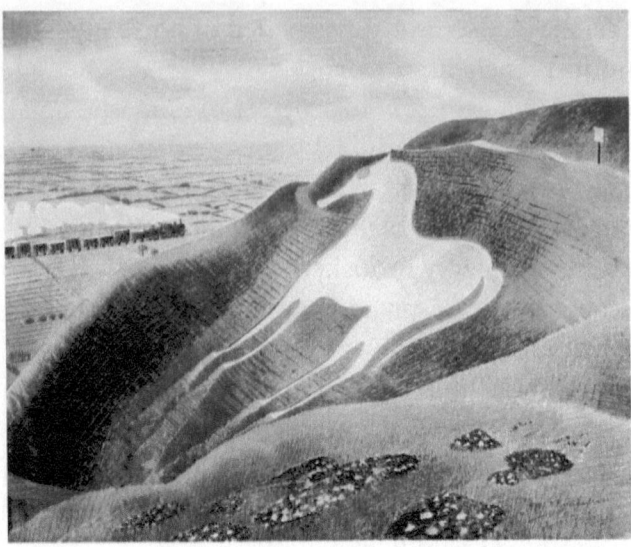

Figure 36. The White Horse was cut into this hillside in Wiltshire, possibly during the late Bronze Age, although it was re-cut in the eighteenth century. Courtesy: visitwiltshire.co.uk.

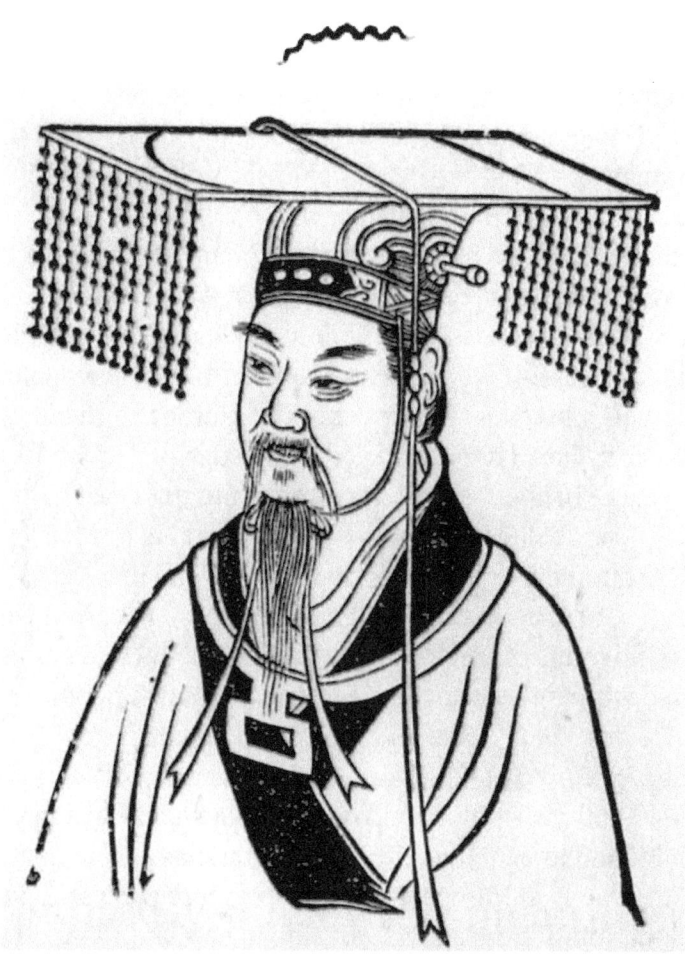

THE YELLOW EMPEROR: *BORRELIA* IN CHINA

Figure 37. *The Inner Canon of the Yellow Emperor or Esoteric Scripture of the Yellow Emperor*, is an ancient Chinese medical text that has been the fundamental doctrinal source for Traditional Chinese Medicine for more than two millennia. The work is composed of two texts, each of eighty-one chapters or treatises in a question-and-answer format between Huang Di, the mythical Yellow Emperor and six of his equally legendary ministers. Woodcut, 1100 AD.

The discovery of a hoard of human teeth in a Chinese cave shows that Early Modern Humans had reached South China more than 80,000 years ago. This early date contrasts with their arrival in Europe at 45,000 years ago, suggesting that it took tens of thousands of years longer for humans to populate Europe than China. When Homo sapiens emerged from Africa about 100,000 years ago they swept eastward with little resistance from other hominid species. But when they headed north, they encountered Neanderthals who had already controlled Europe for hundreds of thousands of years. Humans stayed at the edge of Europe for 40,000 years. In contrast, the migration's progress eastward was rapid. It is possible that an early wave of migrants headed eastwards through Arabia away from Europe and that the colonization of Europe through the Middle East occurred via later waves of migrants. Along the way, Early Modern Humans also interacted with the Denisovans. All modern human populations in Asia include a small percentage of Archaic humans genes (Dennell, 2015).

    A 40,000-year-old individual from Tianyuan Cave in China, has been found to be to more related to present-day and ancient Asians than he is to Europeans, but shares more alleles with a 35,000-year-old European individual than he shares with other ancient Europeans, indicating that the separation between early Europeans and early Asians was not a single population split. The Tianyuan individual shares more alleles with some Native American groups in South America than with Native Americans elsewhere, providing further support for a population substructure in Asia that persisted from 40,000 years ago until the colonization of the Americas. This study of the Tianyuan individual highlights the complex migration and subdivision of early human populations in Eurasia (Hu, 2009).

    Investigation of East Asian Y haplotypes supports the existence of demographic expansions toward East Asia via a northern route, which started between fifteen and eighteen thousand years ago, following the Last Glacial Maximum. However, the demographic input via the northern route is mostly restricted to North East Asian populations and contributed limited

Y chromosomes to current East Asian populations. Among them, haplogroup Q-M242 and R-M207 likely represent the earliest settlers via the northern route. In addition, it was confirmed that the Paleolithic colonization of East Asia via a southern route made a substantial contribution to the extant East Asian Y chromosome gene pool. Paleolithic migrations shaped a south-to-north clonal structure, with postglacial migrations via the northern route enlarging the genetic divergence between Souther and Northern China. The study of Y chromosome data, primarily from Y haplogroup O, C, and D (Su et al. 1999; Shi et al. 2005; Shi et al. 2008; Zhong et al. 2010), suggests that the southern route made a substantial contribution to the early peopling of East Asia, which was also supported by the phylogeography of Y haplogroup N-M231 (Rootsi et al. 2007). Q1a1-M120 and Q1a3-M346 are the two major sub-lineages of Y-haplogroup Q. Q1a1-M120 is an East Asian specific sub-haplogroup. It also occurs in most North East Asian populations.

In South East Asian populations, Q occurs mainly in Southern Han Chinese with relatively low diversity, implying that the spread of Q1a1-M120 was from north to south likely due to the demic-diffusion of Han culture during Neolithic times (Wen, Li, et al. 2004). Notably, Q1a3*-M346 is the ancestral Y haplogroup of Q1a3a-M3, which occurs only in Native American populations (Bortolini et al. 2003; Zegura et al. 2004; Karafet et al. 2008). The trace of Q1a3*-M346 in the North East Asian populations provides important evidence in supporting the proposed prehistoric migration from Central Asia to the Americas. Collectively, the phylogeographic structure of Y haplogroup Q reveals early demographic expansions via northern Eurasia. New finds are also forcing a re-examination of old Chinese books that describe historical or legendary figures of great height, with deep-set blue or green eyes, long noses, full beards, and red or blond hair that now seem accurate (Mallory & Mair, 2000).This was the Yamnaya migration.

Southern China and/or Southeast Asia likely served as a refuge and source post-Last Glacial Maximum dispersal(s). The detailed dissection of Y haplogroup M revealed the existence of an

inland dispersal in mainland East Asia during the post-glacial period. It was this dispersal that expanded not only to western China but also to northeast India and to the south Himalaya region. A similar phylogeographic distribution pattern was also observed for Y haplogroup F1c. This inland post-glacial dispersal was in agreement with the spread of the Mesolithic culture originating in South China and northern Vietnam (Peng, Min-Sheng,et al., 2011)

The Y haplogroups O, C, D, N, and Q are common in East Eurasians, and the Y haplogroups J, G, and R are common in West Eurasians. All the strongly expanding Y chromosomal haplogroups had already migrated to East Asia more than twenty thousand years before their Neolithic expansion, thus supporting a boom of local farmers in China. This is consistent with the independent origin of agriculture there. The first major population expansions in China, as shown by a mitochondrial tree (among which are also several star-shaped expansions), occurred in the late Paleolithic Age. The earliest agriculture in North China emerged before 10,000 BP. It has been found that three mtDNA clades are present with high frequency across many extant East Asian populations and encompass more than forty percent of the present Han Chinese.

China was one of the few areas in the Northern Hemisphere to maintain temperate forest during the last glacial maxima, so it is likely that *Ixodes* ticks and *Borrelia* also found refuge there. Because of this, the Chinese may have more experience at treating Lyme Disease.The most commonly observed human tick-borne diseases in China today include Lyme Disease, tick-borne encephalitis (Forest encephalitis), Crimean-Congo hemorrhagic fever (Xinjiang hemorrhagic fever), Q-fever, and tularemia. In recent years, some emerging tick-borne diseases, such as *anaplasmosis* and a novel *bunyavirus* infection have been reported in China. Other tick-borne diseases that are not as frequently reported in China include *Rickettsia* and *Babesia*.

Although it is an ancient affliction, Lyme disease was first 'discovered' in China in 1985 in a reforested region of Hailin, Heilongjiang (Meng, 2004). The peak incidence of Lyme Disease occurs from June to August. Its main vectors are *Ixodes persulcatus* ticks in Northern China, *Ixodes granulatus* and

Ixodes sinensis in Southern China, and occasionally *Haemaphysalis bispinosa*. Human cases of Lyme disease have been confirmed in tweety nine provinces.

The major endemic areas in China are the forests of North China. In Heilongjiang, Jilin, Liaoning, and Inner Mongolia, over three million people suffer tick bites annually and approximately 30,000 people become infected with Lyme Disease. Approximately ten percent of the new cases turn into chronic infections over two to seventeen years without treatment (Wang, 2011). It was reported that the serological positivity for Lyme disease in 30,000 people randomly sampled was a mean positivity rate of 5.06% overall and the morbidity was 1.16 to 4.51% in the forests (Hein S, etal., 2012). Tick-borne Encephalitis is an acute infectious disease of the nervous system caused by a virus (TBEV). In China, TBEV was first observed in 1942, and TBEV was first isolated from ticks in 1952.

There is wide dissemination of tick-borne diseases throughout China today. Ticks of numerous species are widely distributed, with diverse living habits and numerous hosts, including birds, reptiles, and mammals. The vast territory, complex geography, climate variability, and diverse ecological environments in China provide various habitats for ticks. Rapid development of international and inter- regional exchange has created favorable conditions for the spread of tick-borne diseases in modern China. The endemic area of tick-borne disease is gradually expanding along with changes and ecological damage to the forest environment (Wu,et al, 2013).

In the past, China has undergone dramatic deforestation. When agriculture became intensive, the majority of the human "work" shifted from food collection to food production. Harvesting domesticated crops constituted a more stable food source and created an intensely modified landscape. This affected the risk of tick-borne infections in China, lowering it. As in Europe and the Americas, the skeletal remains of hunter-gatherers in China display more bone infections and agriculturalists suffered less joint damage (Inoue, 2001).

Three legendary characters have been regarded as the founders of Chinese medicine. The earliest is Fu Xi, who is the legendary figure most associated with the development of acupuncture. The second is Shen Nong, the DivineHusbandry Man, associated with farming, who discovered the curative virtues of herbs by tasting different varieties. The third is Huang Di, the Yellow Emperor, who was said to have written down the dialogue about medicine, including acupuncture, with his ministers and who was credited with having made nine kinds of acupuncture needles. These legends reflect, to a certain extent, the historical facts of the early origins of Chinese medicine and the focus on acupuncture and herbal remedies (Ma, 2000).

Archaeological evidence shows that during the Neolithic Period in China, a kind of polished and sharpened stone called "Bian Shi" (stone needle), defined as "a kind of stone used for treating illnesses by pricking the body"was developed.With the introduction of metallurgy from the west, especially during the period of the Warring States (475-221 BC), metal needles came to be widely used in acupuncture. Nine acupuncture needles were unearthed from the tomb of Prince Liu Sheng of Zong Shan and his wife, of the Western Han Dynasty. They had been buried in the year 89 AD. The needles were made of both silver and gold (Zhang, D., 2007, 155-57).

By the time The Yellow Emperor texts were written, acupuncture had developed into a special branch of Chinese medicine. These writing include many references to acupuncture. The other important manual for acupuncture dates to the eleventh century. Wang Weiyi (circa 987-1067) had the idea of casting statues in bronze where the 657 known acupuncture points were engraved. He wrote a manual to accompany the sculptures called the Illustrated Manual of the Bronze Man Showing Acupuncture and Moxibustion Points [moxibustion involves burning or 'cupping' mugwort, also known as artemesia, instead of inserting needles on specific points on the body](Ma, 2000).

Historic records note that the practice of acupuncture spread out from China, especially into Japan. Texts point to a seventeenth century introduction in the west. The

practice may have actually spread along trading routes through Eurasia much earlier. It has been suggested that Ötzi, an ice mummy with Lyme disease found in the Italian Alps, may have had little tattoos placed on various points or meridians of his body to facilitate either acupuncture or some sort of cupping procedure. Cupping is still a traditional practice in Italy (Osborne, 2015).

China has suffered from numerous epidemics over time. This depleted the population. By 1200 AD, the Chinese total population had grown to more than 120 million, but a 1393 census found only 65 million Chinese surviving. Some of that missing population died from famine and warfare, especially during the transition from the Yuan to Ming rule, but many millions more died of Bubonic Plague. Only people with immune systems, especially those with specific TLR types that could attack and kill that bacteria, survived.

The 1331 plague outbreak began when the Mongols ruled over China. Three years later, the disease had killed over ninety percent of the Hebei Province's population, with deaths totaling over five million people. Archaeological excavations on the shores of Issyk Kul, a lake in what is now in Kyrgyzstan, reveal that the Nestorian Christian trading community there was ravaged by Bubonic Plague in 1338 and 1339. Issyk Kul was a major Silk Road depot and has sometimes been cited as the origin point for the Black Death in Europe. It is a prime habitat for marmots, which carried a virulent form of the disease.

In 1344, the Mongolian Golden Horde attempted to recapture the Crimean port city of Kaffa from the Genoese traders who had seized the town in the late 1200s. A Mongol siege lasted until 1347, when reinforcements brought in from further east introduced the plague to the Mongol troops. Gabriele de Mussis recorded what happened next: "The whole army was affected by a disease which overran the Tartars (Mongols) and killed thousands upon thousands every day." He goes on to charge that the Mongol leader "ordered corpses to be placed in catapults and lobbed into the city in hopes that the intolerable stench would kill everyone inside." This incident is often cited as the first instance of biological warfare in recorded history.

Gilles li Muisis, notes that a "calamitous disease befell the Tartar army, and the mortality was so great and widespread that scarcely one in twenty of them remained alive." The siege of Kaffa produced refugees that fled on ships bound for Genoa. These refugees were the likely primary source for the epidemic of Black Death that went on to decimate Europe. The most significant political impact that the Black Death had on China was that it destroyed the Mongol Empire (Wheelis, 2002). The most important biological impact is that it changed the immune systems of the Chinese, allowing particular sets of genes to survive. It also influenced Chinese Traditional Medical practices.

The Inner Canon of the Yellow Emperor or Esoteric Scripture of the Yellow Emperor is an ancient Chinese medical text that has been the fundamental doctrinal source for Traditional Chinese Medicine for more than two thousand years. The work is composed of two texts, each of eighty-one chapters or treatises in a question-and-answer format between the mythical Yellow Emperor and six of his equally legendary ministers.

The literature of Traditional Chinese Medicine includes treatments for spirochetal diseases. The treatments that were developed were also probably used to treat ancient cases of Lyme Disease, which was recognized as an illness that presented with a combined arthritic/neurological character. According to Traditional Chinese medicine, arthritis is an "impediment disease" which refers to a group of diseases resulting from "invasion of wind, cold, and dampness (Hou, 2015). Some of the herbs recommended for its treatment include *Rhizoma Arisaematis,* a Chinese herb still used to treat Bell's palsy, hemiplegia, convulsions in children, tetanus, and epilepsy, and *Radix Aconiti,* used for facial paralysis, joint pain, gout, inflammation, certain heart problems (pericarditis), fever and skin diseases. Also used was *Flos Caryophylli (clove flower bud)* which is antimicrobial. Its essential oil extracts kill bacteria and *Candida albicans* (Cosentino, et al, 1999, Deans & Ritchie, 1987).

After a deadly plague epidemic in Manchuria at the turn of the Twentieth Century was contained by mandating cremation and applying western plague control techniques, a new medical system

began to emerge in China. The pharmacological effects of the traditional remedies were analyzed and intermeshed with some aspects of western medicine. This integration created a Modern Chinese Medicine (Benedict, 1996).

There is the wide dissemination of tick-borne diseases throughout China exist. First, ticks of numerous species are widely distributed, with diverse living habits and numerous hosts, including birds, reptiles, and mammals. Secondly, the vast territory, complex geography, climate variability, and diverse ecological environments in China provide various habitats for ticks. Thirdly, the rapid development of international and inter-regional exchange has created favorable conditions for the spread of tick-borne diseases. Finally, the epidemic area of tick-borne disease is gradually expanding along with changes and ecological damage to the forest environment.

Chinese herbal remedies have been found to be effective when used to treat Lyme disease (Zhang, 2006). Some were used successfully in treating syphilis, a sexually transmitted disease caused by the spirochete *Treponema pallidum*. Europeans brought this disease to Calcutta in 1498, and by 1520 it had reached Africa and China. The historical use of the name "Cantonese Sores" (*guangdong chuang*) to describe syphilis supports the theory that its spread through China followed the trade routes that linked early European traders with the Canton province. By the 1940's, Syphilis had become a major epidemic within China. When the Communist Party took over, it made the disease a high priority and launched a campaign to abolish it. It was estimated that five percent of the population in large cities carried the disease. The campaign consisted of screening, free treatment, and a crack down on prostitution – a major factor for the spread of the disease. By 1964, Syphilis was a rarity and the infection was nearly eliminated (Hesketh,et al., 2008).

The anti-spirochetal Chinese herbs that were successfully used for treating syphilis are also used for Lyme disease. *Smilax glabrae Rhizoma* is a major ingredient of herbal Lyme formulas. Allicin, the active ingredient of garlic, decanoylacetaldehyde, an active ingredient of *Houttuyniae Herba,* Coptin, an active

ingredient of *Coptis chinensis Radix* and *Scutellariae Radix* are all used to kill spirochetes.

Early stages of spirochetal infection are also treated by the formulas used in the *Shang Han Lun:* Isatis leaf, Smilax, Isatis root, Gardenia, Andrographis, Hu-chang, Chien-li-kuang and Scute are mentioned. These herbs have broad-spectrum antibiotic and antiviral properties. The book *Thousand Formulas and Thousand Herbs of Traditional Chinese Medicine* delineate six herbs that can be used to clear infection. They have been found to heal *Leptospirosis, Treponema denticola* (spirochetes in oral flora), *Bartonella* and many gram negative and gram positive bacteria. Xu Duan (Chinese Teasel Root) is taken to help drive spirochetes from the joints into the blood stream where they can be killed by other herbs. *Reishi* mushroom and *Astragalus* are also mentioned (Buhner, 2012, Zhang, 2006).

When Traditional Chinese Medicine formularies have been subjected to scientific testing, some have been found to be effective against *Borrelia* and co-infections. *Houttuynia* is effective against *Bartonella*. Five traditional essential oils (oregano, cinnamon bark, clove bud, citronella, and wintergreen) at a low concentration showed high anti-persister cell activity that was comparable to the drug daptomycin. Interestingly, some highly active essential oils were found to also have excellent anti-biofilm ability, as shown by their ability to dissolve aggregated biofilm-like structures. These include oregano, cinnamon bark, and clove bud (Feng et al , 2017). Because of their extensive history with spirochetal diseases, Chinese herbal medicine can be a helpful augmentation for combating Lyme disease.

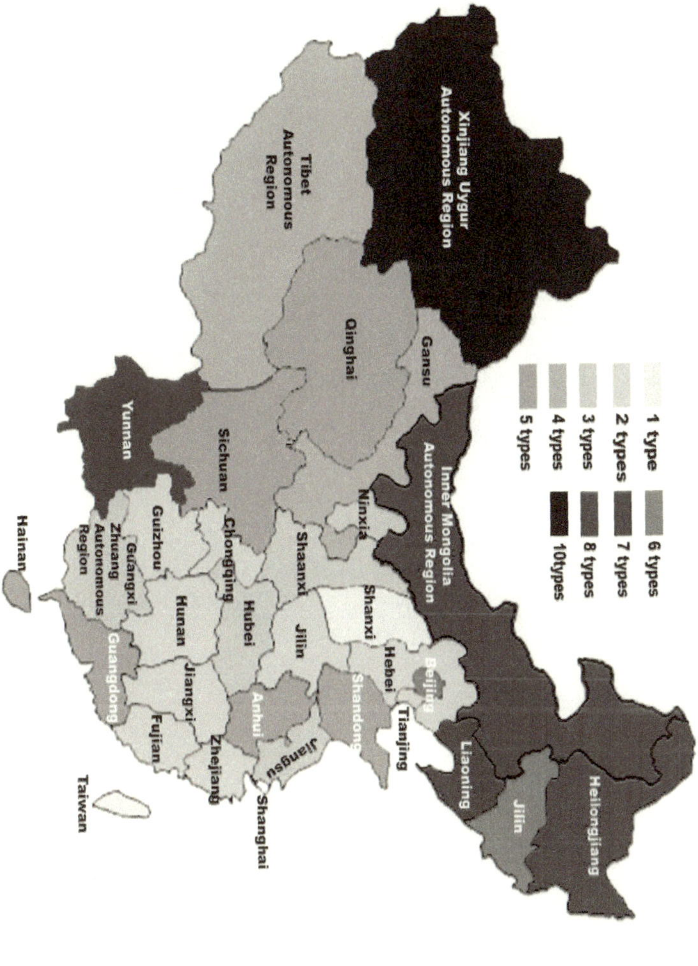

Figure 38. Distribution of Tick-borne Infections in China (Wu, et al., 2013).

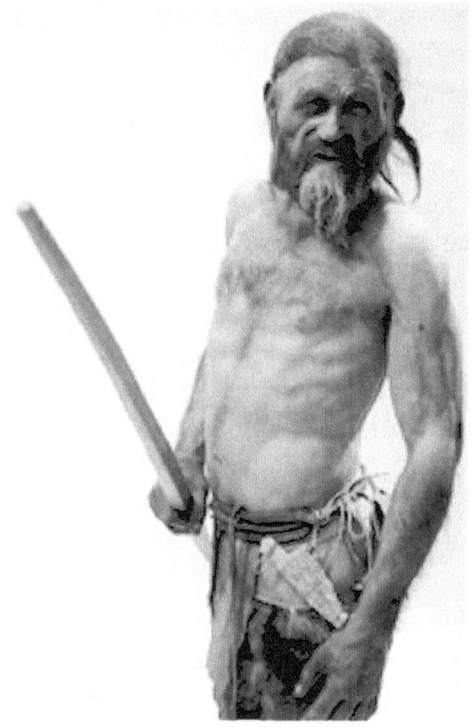

Figure 39. Sculpture of Ötzi as he may have appeared in life. Courtesy: South Tyrol Museum of Archaeology, Bolzano, Italy.

ÖTZI: BORRELIA ON ICE

Ötzi is the name given to the oldest known European mummy. He was just forty five years old when he died from hypothermia and excessive blood loss around 5,300 years ago. He died at a time when Europe was undergoing a climatic cool down and was buried by ice quite soon after his death. He may also be one of the most studied mummies in existence. We know quite a lot about him. He spent his childhood near the present village of Feldthurns, north of Bolzano, Italy but later went to live in a valley about 50 km further north. He spent his entire life within a 37-mile range south of where he came to his final rest after being shot with an arrow. Öttzi was about 5 foot, 3 inches tall and weighed 110 pounds. He had brown eyes, type "O" blood, Y haplotype G, was lactose intolerant, and was pre-disposed to heart disease (Fowler, 2001). Ötzi also suffered from the earliest documented case of Lyme Disease infection. Although scientists don't really know how sick Ötzi was during his lifetime, the discovery of sixty percent of a *Borrelia* genome within his Neolithic body confirms that this pathogen has plagued humans for thousands of years (Keller, et al, 2012). We also know that Neolithic people treated various illnesses with various herbal remedies. Ötzi was carrying with him a form of mushroom that is know to have antibiotic qualities (Caprasso, 1998).

Ötzi lived his life at the edge of the forest in an early agrarian village but he also hunted wild animals in his alpine environment. By examining the proportions of his tibia, femur and pelvis, it has been determined that Ötzi's lifestyle included long walks over hilly terrain. This degree of mobility is not characteristic of other Copper Age Europeans suggesting that Ötzi was a high-altitude shepherd. The clothes of the world's oldest intact human mummy suggest the Iceman lived in a relatively advanced farming society. He wore a goat and sheepskin coat, goatskin leggings, grass matting in his shoes and a sheepskin loincloth. Genetic analysis shows that his arrow quiver was made from roe deer skin, while his fur hat was fashioned from the genetic ancestors of the brown bears that are still seen in the Alpine region today. He trod a landscape that was also inhabited by *Borrelia* laden *Ixodid ricinus* ticks. This forested geographical area is now located between Italy and Austria and still has one of the highest modern Lyme disease infection rates in all of Europe. Roe deer, *Capreolus capreolus,* are considered reservoir species for both *Borrelia* and *Rickettsia* and are important blood meal hosts for feeding ticks.

We know a bit about what Ötzi ate by examining what was included in his stomach contents. He had eaten two meals that day- both with meat, including a fine slice or two of processed bacon most likely dried and cured goat meat. Both were consumed with some grain-einkorn wheat and barley. Seeds from flax and poppy were consumed, as well as kernels of sloes (small plumlike fruits of the blackthorn tree) and various seeds of berries. He had also eaten pollen with the first meal that showed that it had been

consumed in a mid-altitude conifer forest and other pollens indicated the presence of wheat and legumes, which may have been from domesticated crops. Pollen grains of hop-hornbeam were also discovered. The pollen was very well preserved, with the cells inside remaining intact, indicating that it had been fresh (a few hours old) at the time of Ötzi's death, which places the event in the spring. Einkorn wheat is harvested in the late summer and sloes in the autumn, so these must have been stored from the previous year (Rollo et al., 2002).

High levels of copper particles and arsenic were found in Ötzi's hair. This, along with a copper axe made from 99.7% pure copper, has led scientists to speculate that Ötzi was involved in copper smelting. His copper axe had a yew handle, he had a flint-bladed knife with an ash handle, an antler tool, and a quiver of 14 arrows with viburnum and dogwood shafts. He also had a type of tinder fungus in what appeared to be a fire starting kit (Bower, July 2017).

Ötzi had sixty one tattoos, some of which were located to in places that coincide with acupuncture points that are used coincide to treat the symptoms of diseases like digestive parasites, Lyme disease, and osteoarthrosis. Some scientists believe that these tattoos indicate an early type of acupuncture. Ötzi had several tattoos made by rubbing fire soot mixed with glittering stone crystals, into small cuts including groups of short, parallel, vertical lines to both sides of the lumbar spine, a cruciform mark behind the right knee, and various marks around both ankles. Radiological examination of his bones showed "age-conditioned or strain-induced degeneration" in these areas, including osteochondrosis and slight spondylosis in the lumbar spine, wear-and-tear degeneration in the knee, and especially the ankle joints. It has been speculated that these tattoos may have been related to pain relief treatments similar to acupressure or acupuncture. If so, this is at least 2000 years before their previously known earliest documented use in China (c. 1000 BCE)(MSNBC - July 17, 2009).

Mitochondrial DNA analysis has shown that the *Borrelia* bacteria had found its way deep into Ötzi's bones and that he had suffered from bone loss as a result of his infection. This discovery has led to research into the effects of Lyme disease on bones. Bone

pain has been reported since Lyme disease was discovered. One study has found that untreated Lyme bacteria cause significant bone loss in the longer bones of mice mere weeks after infection. The amount of bone loss was directly correlated to the bacterial load found in the bones (Moriarity, T., December 8, 2016).

    A clinical musculoskeletal examination of Ötzi demonstrated arthritis and other forms of long-term musculoskeletal damage. Several musculoskeletal abnormalities have been identified on X-ray and CAT scans (Gostner & Vigl, 2002). These include osteoarthritis of the facet joints of the neck, and osteoarthritis of the right hip. Musculoskeletal symptoms in Lyme disease include tendon and bursal pain, and migratory joint pains and swelling, especially in the knees. About sixty percent of untreated patients develop chronic arthritis, and about ten percent develop cartilage damage and bone erosions (Steere et al. 1987). Whether Ötzi was symptomatic at any time in his life with some or several manifestations of Lyme disease cannot be known, but his right knee and right ankle show cartilage damage which may be attributed to the fact that he was infected with Lyme disease (Kean, et al., February 2013).

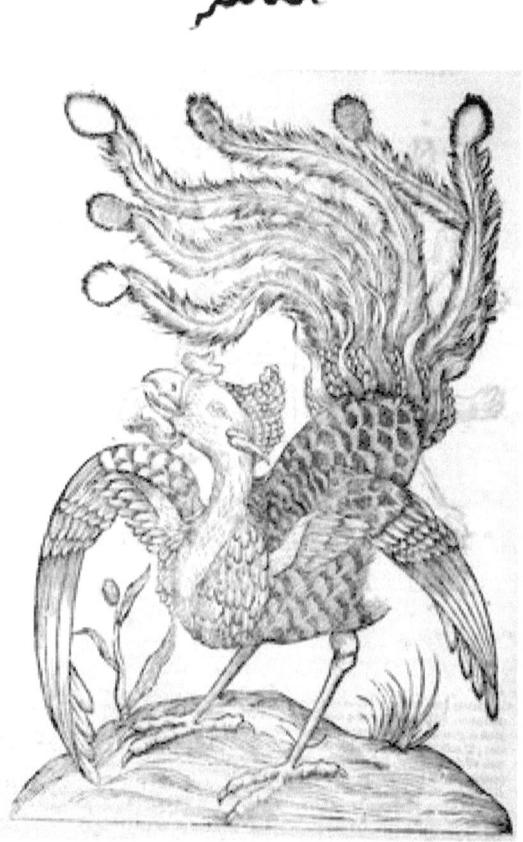

Figure 40. Woodcut of *Gallus Indicus auritus tridactylus* by Aldronvandi, 1570

CHICKEN! BORRELIA FOR THE BIRDS!

Although all *Borrelia* share a great deal of genomic features, some have developed into very host specific pathogens. *Borrelia anserinas*, known as avian spirochaetosis, is exclusive to poultry- the descendants of dinosaurs (Fukunaga,et al.1996). It infects turkeys, chickens, pheasants, ducks, geese, or birds. *Borrelia anserina* is found on a worldwide basis. There have been no documented cases of human infection with *Borrelia anserina* and the ticks responsible for spreading avian spirochaetosis are not thought to seek human blood meal hosts. The bacterium is transmitted from bird to bird by soft ticks in the *Argas* and *Ornitodorus* genera. The major symptoms of birds with an infection of *Borrelia anserina* are: anemia, diarrhea, and severe

neurological dysfunctions. Outbreaks of the disease tend to occur during peak tick activity.

Borrelia anserinas is thought to have speciated among wild birds in Southeast Asia or India, and to have been spread to its current world wide endemic status through chicken domestication. It was carried out of Asia during the process by which domesticated chickens were spread throughout the world . Scientists have identified three closely related species that might have bred to produce the modern chicken. Chickens (*Gallus domestics*) were first domesticated from a wild form called red junglefowl (*Gallus gallus*), a bird that still runs wild[it does very little flying] in Southeast Asia. It was naturally hybridized with the gray junglefowl (*Gallus sonneratii)*of India which gave it yellow skin. That occurred probably between eight and ten thousand years ago.

Chickens were spread through the introduction and popularity of the cultural practice of cock fighting and not as a particularly important food source (Sawai,et al. 2010). Chickens became a sacred animal in some cultures. They arrived in Egypt in 1750 BC as fighting birds and additions to exotic menageries. Artistic depictions of the bird adorned royal tombs. Yet, it would be another 1,000 years before the bird became a popular commodity for eating among ordinary Egyptians.

The prodigious and ever-watchful hen is a worldwide symbol of nurturance and fertility. Eggs were hung in Egyptian temples to ensure a bountiful river flood. The lusty rooster became a signifier of virility but also, in the ancient Persian faith of Zoroastrianism, a benign spirit that crowed at dawn to herald the turning point in the cosmic struggle between darkness and light. For the Romans, chickens were fortunetellers- especially in wartime. Chickens accompanied Roman armies and their behavior was observed before battle- a good appetite meant victory was likely. Chickens became a delicacy among the Romans, whose culinary innovations included the omelet and the practice of stuffing birds for cooking. Archaeological digs have uncovered chicken bones from about 800 B.C. in Europe. The chicken's status appears to have diminished with the collapse of Rome. In the post-Roman period,

the size of chickens returned to what it was during the Iron Age. As the centuries went by, hardier fowls such as geese and partridge were favored on medieval tables (Lawlor &Adler, 2012).

Gallus gallus may have spread from Southeast Asia, traveling either north to China and southwest to India or there may have been multiple domestication events in distinct areas of South and Southeast Asia, southern China, Thailand, Burma, and India. Genetic studies hint at strongly hybrid genomes. The earliest archaeological evidence for domesticated chickens to date is from China at about 5400 BC(Xiang et al. 2014). Domesticated chickens appear in the Indus Valley by about 2000 BC and, from there the chicken spread into Europe and Africa. Chickens arrived in the Middle East starting with Iran at 3900 BC, followed by Turkey and Syria (2400-2000 BC) and into Jordan by 1200 BC.The earliest firm evidence for chickens in East Africa are illustrations from several sites in New Kingdom Egypt. Chickens were introduced into western Africa multiple times, arriving at Iron Age sites by the first millennium AD. Chickens arrived in the southern Levant about 2500 BC and in Iberia about 2000 BC (Dueppen, 2011).

In 2004, the first complete map of a chicken genome was produced. The genome map provided an excellent opportunity to study how millennia of domestication can alter a species. The researchers found important mutations in a gene designated TBC1D1, which regulates glucose metabolism and is associated with obesity. Another mutation that resulted from selective breeding is in the TSHR (thyroid-stimulating hormone receptor) gene. In wild animals this gene coordinates reproduction with day length, confining egg laying to specific seasons. The mutation disabling this gene enables chickens to lay eggs all year long (Hillier, et al., 2004).

Some archaeologists believe that chickens were first introduced to the New World by Polynesians who reached the Pacific coast of South America a century or so before Columbus sailed the blue in 1492. While it was assumed that they had been brought to the Americas by the Spanish conquistadors, pre-Columbian chickens have been identified at several sites throughout the Americas prior to Spanish colonization.

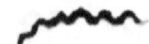

Radiocarbon dates from South American sites fall as early as 1350. Likely genetic markers of authentic ancient Polynesian chickens have been found in South America. Chickens were transported from New Guinea into Micronesia by about 3,850 years ago; and separately from New Guinea to the Solomon Islands, Vanuatu ,and eastward at a later date. (Dueppen, 2011).

Among Polynesian chickens, one particular cluster of mitochondrial DNA, Haplogroup D, is the signature of the founding lineage. Haplogroup E is the key piece of genetic evidence supporting the pre-Columbian presence of chickens on the coast of South America.: Haplogroup E has been found on Easter Island and on coastal Chile. Researchers have found that Haplogroup D closely follows the distribution of cockfighting in India, Indonesia, China, and Japan, and it was also a traditional practice in Polynesian societies. In contrast, the other haplogroups, including A, B, and E, are ubiquitous worldwide (Storey, 2013). When chickens were transported around the world, *Borrelia aseninia* seem to have gone along for the ride, spreading along with the chickens!

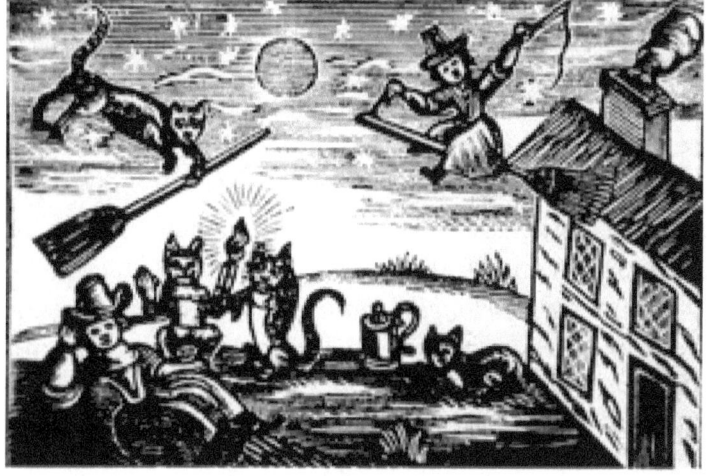

Figure 41. Anonymous, unknown date, woodcut. From "1000 Quaint Cuts from Books of Other Days," *The Strand Magazine*, 1892, p. 206.

ROMANS, CATS, AND BARTONELLA!

"The major killers of humanity throughout our recent history are infectious diseases that evolved from diseases of animals....Because diseases have been the biggest killers of people, they have also been decisive shapers of history."

Jared Diamond.

Humans and cats, after eying each other from afar for eons, started living with each other about 12,000 years or so ago when cats became domesticated. The last common ancestor of both wild cats and domesticated cats (*Felis catus*) lived more than 100,000 years ago in the Middle East. A 2007 research project found that the cat first emerged as a domesticated species at about the same time that dogs, sheep, and goats were also being domesticated. There also seems to have been separate and independent domestication events in Egypt and China. Since then, domesticated cats have spread around the world in the company of humans, sometimes being transported on boats (Ottoni, et al., June 19, 2017).

Cats helped spread the tick-borne co-infection *Bartonella henselae* as they moved around the world. Humans are an incidental host. The cat is a natural reservoir for this bacteria. Approximately 12 species of Bartonella can infect humans and animals (Maguina,2001). *Bartonella* dates back 16-68,000 years. Cats may have introduced the bacteria into Northern Europe. DNA of *Bartonella henselae,* which causes Cat-Scratch Fever in humans, has been found in an 800 year old cat tooth from France (La et al, 2004). Vectors for *Bartonella quintana,* also called Trench Fever because of its prevalence during WWI, include ticks, lice and fleas.

DNA of *Bartonella quintana* has been found in a 4,000 year old human tooth from Roaix in southern France (Drancourt, M, 2005). Trench Fever is another ancient bacterial disease that has only been recognized for a short time. It's case history is only about a century old. However, *Bartonella quintana* is one of the most common infectious organisms found in ancient human DNA. Once thought of as a self-limiting moderate 'five-day' fever, it is now known that it can cause endocarditis and chronic bacteremia. After the chance discovery of Trench Fever in captive macaques that were being transported in both directions between the United States and China, the extent of *Bartonella quintana* in macaques in primate centers in China was studied. Blood samples from macaques at four geographically distant primate centers were collected. They found that the *Bartonella quintana* from all four centers had enough genetic diversity to suggest multiple sources originating in the wild . By multi-locus sequence typing (MLST), a type of genetic fingerprinting, they found more genetic diversity just in the macaques from these centers than from all human isolates analyzed to date around the world. This suggests that macaques are the likely original host population of this form of the ancient zoonosis (Sato, 2015).

An early cat skeleton placed in a grave dating to 11,500 BP has been found on the Mediterranean island of Cyprus. By 7,000 BC, cats were co-habitating with humans in China, where legend entrusts them with the important task of keeping time and distributing luck. When they were domesticated in Egypt by around 4,000 years ago, they hit the lottery. The Egyptian culture

revered cats as sacred. The goddess Bastet, commonly depicted as a cat or as a woman with a cat's head, was among the most popular deities of the Egyptians. She was the keeper of hearth and home, protector of women's secrets, guardian against evil spirits and disease, and the goddess of cats. The very name `cat' derives from the North African word "quattah"(Morris, 175). The colloquial word for a cat - `puss' or `pussy' derives from another name for Bastet, Pasht.

Cats may have been brought to the Italian peninsula by Phoenician traders who smuggled them out of Egypt and had started the practice of keeping cats on ships to control vermin. Cats are depicted in a 1st century AD mosaic from Pompeii's *House of the Faun* [now located at the Pompeii Archaeological Museum in Naples].

When the Romans went northward to conquer Gaul and Britannia, they brought cats with them as grain storage guardians. Cats joined the Roman Legions and traveled with them wherever they would go. The cats were rewarded with human companionship and all of the mice that they could possibly eat. Cats made their way across Europe with the Romans. An excavation of the Ancient Roman Fort at Bothwellhaugh in Scotland found solid evidence of domestic cats cohabiting with the soldiers. Paw prints from domestic cats have been found pressed into at least four clay tiles. The fort was built in around 142 A.D. Although cat bones have been found at a small number of Iron Age sites in Britain, early cat skeletons are most often found in association with Roman archaeological sites. Roman colonial families were avid cat owners. Roman cats may have strayed and interbred with *Felis Silvestris,* the wild cat that was at that time still common across the higher land of Britain and Western Europe. In the Fourth Century AD, when the Romans retreated back to Rome, they left behind a lot of cats in France and Britain (Faure & Kitchner, 2009).

During the process of converting Europe to Christianity, as the Roman Catholic Church worked to stamp out paganism, animal worship, and all other non-Christian beliefs, cats became a target. Then Europe went Crusading! Nine Crusades were launched between 1095 and 1291, mostly to try to recapture Jerusalem from the Muslims. Domestic crusades were also launched against groups or individuals throughout Europe who were considered dangerous to the church or its teachings. Medieval people became obsessed with the devil and believed that he and his servants could assume human and/or animal forms. The cat was the domesticated animal most closely associated with paganism and their time in Egypt with the goddess Bastet came back to haunt them. Cats came under suspicion.

Unlike dogs, cats do not behave subserviently toward humans. They are also very active at night and engage in loud, raucous mating rituals-attributes that would soon be applied to witches. In the early thirteenth century Pope Gregory IX declared in a Papal Bull Vox in Rama that a sect had been caught worshipping the black cat, which he called a "Vessel of the Devil." This led to attacks on cats and cat burnings. By the beginning of the fourteenth century, Europe's cat population had been severely depleted. Only wily feral cats survived in many areas. While the cats were away, the rats did play, rodent populations increased, and brought with them fleas and plague!

The *Bubonic Plague* swept via the Mongolian Golden Horde's conquests from China towards Europe, beginning there with the arrival of shiploads of evacuating Genoese merchants. Called the Black Death, it killed twenty-five million Europeans in only three years. Thousands of farm animals died as well, either from the plague or lack of care. It has long been argued that the death of so many cats allowed the Bubonic Plague to become pandemic in Europe. While this theory has been disputed, there seems to be no doubt that a decrease in the cat population would result in an increase in the number of rodents, especially as the abandoned fields and pastures of Europe re-forested (Georgievska, 2017). Cats continued to be exterminated for religious reasons for another three hundred years.

The inhabitants of European nations, believing the cat to in league with the devil, shunned not only the animal but anyone who seemed overly fond of them. In 1485, The Roman Catholic Church affirmed the existence of witches. Elderly women who cared for

cats were especially susceptible to punishment for witchcraft. The Protestant Reformation did little to change the situation. Hatred of cats was non-denominational. England's Witchcraft Act of 1563 associated the keeping of cats with "wickedness" and led to the executions of cats and their owners.The coronation of Queen Elizabeth I in England was celebrated with a massive cat burning ceremony. The English brought these ideas and practices with them when they explored and began to colonize the Americas. As late as 1658 Edward Topsel, in his work on natural history wrote that: the familiars of Witches do most ordinarily appear in the shape of cats, which is an argument that this beast is dangerous to soul and body (Drymon,2008).

Cats spread around the world in waves.The first wave arrived wild from Africa into the Middle East, Eastern Mediterranean, and spread across Eurasia. The ancestor of all modern domesticated cats, *Felis Catus,*alive today on a worldwide basis is the African Wildcat, *Felis silvestris lybica* (Vigne, et al, 2016). Having made their way out of Africa, these cats were domesticated by the earliest farmers during the earliest days of agriculture. Another wave took place thousands of years later as cats from Egypt quickly spread to the rest of Africa and Asia. Their genetic markers have been discovered in cats from Bulgaria, Turkey, and sub Saharan Africa. Cats are featured in Scythian jewelry designs, showing that they had reached the Eurasian steppes at an early date. Cats that shared Egyptian mitochondrial DNA, which is passed down only on the mother's side, have been found as far north as a Viking site in Northern Germany by the eighth and eleventh century (Perrson, 2016).

Cats were also independently domesticated in China. A different species, the leopard cat, *Prionailurus bengalensis,*was living with humans before the domesticated cat arrived in the region.The leopard cat did not, however, persist across time. House cats in China today are descended from the African wildcat, like everywhere else on the planet. The leopard cat survives in Asia as a relatively common wild species (Vigne, J. et al, January 22, 2016).

Cats are celebrated in Chinese mythology and culture. In

China, the cat is considered lucky. Records of the relationship between cats and humans in Chinese history goes back to the time of Confucius (551 – 479 BC). The *Chinese Book of Rites* tells the story of the cat goddess Li Shou. It's a story that teaches a lesson in responsible behavior and explains how humans came to talk and rule over the creatures of the earth.After falling to concentrate on keeping order, Li Shou and the cats were put in charge of keeping time for the earth.Chinese mythology states that you can tell the time of day by looking into a cat's eyes- the pupils of the cat's eyes control the height of the sun above the horizon (Halloway, 2013).

In November, 2013, archaeologists found some new evidence in regards to the domestication of cats at a dig site in the village of Quanhucun, China.The bones were about 5,300 years old.The age of these cats' bones show that cats were being domesticated in China for at least 1,300 years before they were domesticated in Ancient Egypt.The domestication of cats in China must have started with grain stored by Chinese farmers (Yaowu Hu, et al, 2013). Bone fragments belonging to at least two different small cats were found. Two findings from the analysis of the cat bones were particularly interesting: The cats had been eating grain. Isotope analysis of the cats bones showed that there was a significant amount of grain in these cats' diets. Scientists propose that this is evidence of humans feeding the cats from their own grain stores(Driscoll, 2007).

Many modern cats and humans have asymptomatic *Bartonella* or *Bartonella*-like (BLO) infections in their bodies. Veterinarians say that eighty percent of all house cats and nearly one hundred percent of all hunting cats carry the microbes. Fleas and ticks bite the cats and infect them with the *Bartonella*-like organisms, which are then transmitted to humans directly through contact or when they get bitten by fleas and ticks carried in by cats. *Bartonella* and BLO infections are therefore probably the most common of the vector-borne Lyme disease co-infections. Prevalence of the infection varies geographically. In one study of rheumatic patients in a Lyme endemic area, sixty three percent had *Bartonella* antibodies in their blood (Maggi, et al, 2012). *Bartonella henselae* has been found in questing *Ixodes ricinus*

ticks in Europe (Dietrich, et al, 2010). Northern climates reportedly have less prevalence of the disease but some scientists are convinced that *Bartonella* is the stealth cause of many neurological, inflammatory and chronic diseases in humans. Once symptomatic, *Bartonella* is difficult to treat. As one doctor states, "You cannot float humans or horses in enough doxycycline to kill this bacteria."

During early infection, *Bartonella* not only survive but also divide inside immune cells called macrophages, prevent cell death that would normally occur in response to infection, and suppress immune system activation. In a murine[mouse] model, intracellular *Bartonella* use the lymphatic system to enter the bloodstream. and evade the human innate immune system because they are not recognized as a pathogen by the TLR4 once within the macrophages. Once phagocytized, the organisms can avoid destruction (Hong,et al., 2017).

In the human body, *Bartonella* infects the CD 34 that function as important adhesion molecules required for T cells to enter lymph nodes but can also act as molecular Teflon, blocking mast cells, eosinophils and dendritic cell adhesion, causing vascular lesions to appear. The lesions may also be found in a variety of organs including the gastro-intestinal tract where they may cause hematemesis[vomiting of blood](Soucheray, 2013). A vast majority of people with *Bartonella* experience swelling of the glands.

Cat-scratch disease is usually a self-limiting condition in immunocompetent individuals. When combined with Lyme disease, it can be especially virulent. The spectrum of systemic involvement in bartonellosis ranges from endocarditis to thyroiditis, arthritis, haemolytic anemia, and glomerulonephritis (Rattanavong, et al, 2014, Sanchez Clemente, et al.2012, Chaudhry,et al, 2015, Chiuri, et al., 2013). The ocular manifestations of Bartonella spp. infection are likewise myriad and have included retinal artery occlusions (Eiger-Moscovich, et al., 2015), and even a macular hole(Seth,et al., 2016).

Like *Borrelia*, *Bartonella* really gets into your bones (Mirouse, et al., 2015) sometimes causing nodules (bumps) on the forearms and shin bone area. *Bartonella* can cause burning sensations and redness and swelling of the palms and soles of the feet. It can cause large lumps on the face, neck, chest and back. Infections often present with "red streaks" resembling cat scratches forming on the skin. During the time of the great witch hunts, these scratches were called the Mark of the Devil , and were thought to be caused by an attack by preternatural forces (Drymon, 2008).

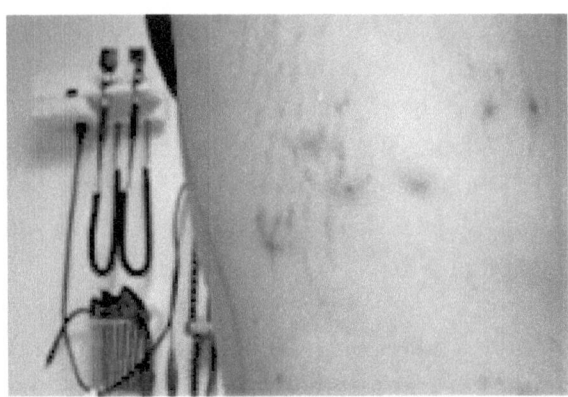

Figure 42. Bartonella rash with 'cat scratches.' Facebook, public posting.

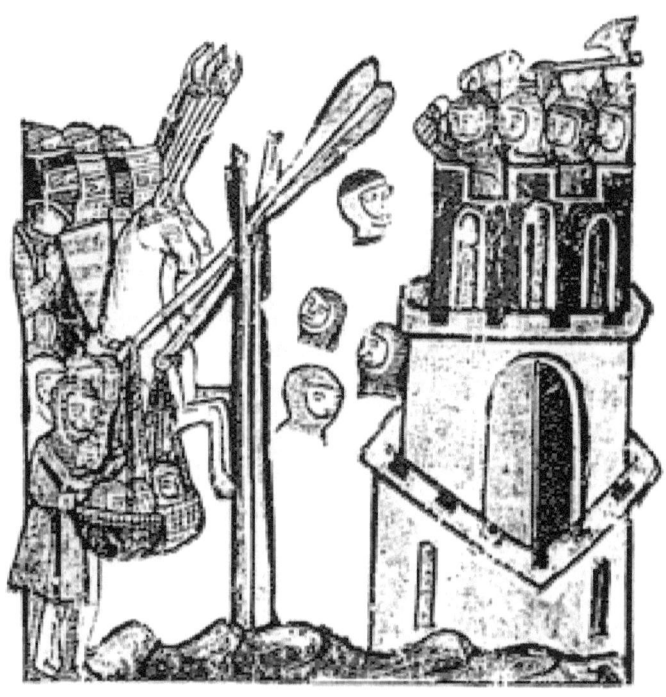

QUESTING FOR CRUSADERS:
BORRELIA IN THE MOUTH

Figure 43. Trebuchet use during a Crusader siege.   13th Century woodcut.

At the Council of Claremont in 1095, Pope Urban II preached the need for a holy war to save Jerusalem from Muslim Invaders. Thousands of Christian warriors immediately began affixing a cross to their garments and carrying flags to become Crusaders. There was an enthusiastic response to Urban's preaching from all classes in Western Europe. Christian volunteers took a public vow and in return they received plenary indulgences from the Church, insuring their fast track to heaven after death. The objective of the first crusade was to reclaim the Holy Land, including Jerusalem,

from Saracen [Muslim] control. Over time the objectives expanded to freeing Spain from the Moors, attacking Cathars, driving Pagans from Eastern Europe, and to acquiring islands in the Mediterranean as part of a set of supply chain ports. In total, there were there were nine crusades. The departure of the first crusade was set for for August 15,1096, to coincide with the Day of the Feast of the Assumption. Various sets of national troops started off and reached the Levant between November and April of 1097(Erbstösser,1978).

This had meant a between three and eight month trip by land and sea that crossed many heavily forested regions in France and Italy. Most Crusaders had to cross some French territory, which at the time consisted of at least fifty percent forest cover (Mather et al., 1999). Some marched through the Alpine region of Italy, only a few miles from the area where Ötzi had grown up four thousand years earlier.

The overland and sea journeys in crowded conditions led to malnutrition, frostbite, drowning, and the spread of communicable diseases acquired from fleas, lice and ticks as well as person to person contact. An individual with an immune system developed for cooler northern Europe might have been at considerable risk migrating to the Middle East. First, they would encounter new diseases to which they would have little immunity. Many suffered from vitamin deficiency and malnutrition, which also weakened their resistance to disease. Moreover, participating in a culture that had developed for a different climatic region would have increased the risk of succumbing to conditions such as heat stroke or food poisoning. Some historians have suggested that only one in twenty Crusaders, barely five percent, who set out survived to even reach the Holy Land. In total, it is estimated that more than 1.7 million people died during the Crusades (Mathews, 2011).

The third crusade, led by of King Richard I of England and Philippe Augustus II of France, started in 1191, but after just a few days of intense fighting before the walls of Acre, both kings fell ill with an illness then known as *arnaldia* or in French *leonardie-* which became better known as Trench Mouth during WWI. Trench mouth is a severe infection of the tooth margins and gums

characterized by painful bleeding gums and ulcers. Although the mouth naturally contains a balance of bacteria, fungi, and viruses, in certain conditions harmful bacteria overgrowth is promoted by poor dental hygiene, poor nutrition, stress, a weakened immune system and/or other infections. It is sometimes confused with the oral symptoms of land scurvy, which is caused by a nutritional deficiency of Vitamin C. Trench Mouth is caused by the symbiotic micro-organisms *Bacillus fusiformis* and the spirochete *Borrelia vincenti*. For weeks Kings Richard and Philippe both seemed close to death but both lived to fight another day (Nicholson, 1997).

Richard's forces had employed one hundred ships carrying eight thousand men from England for France. From France, they had sailed with additional ships, some of which carried beehives along with their beekeepers. On July 11, the English used trebuchets to hurl those hives into the city. The bees were "not at all happy with their treatment so they took their wrath out on the defenders who were even less happy." After the fall of Acre, an epidemic struck the Crusader Army beginning in the summer of 1192. King Richard became ill again– this time with a malady called *asfebris emitritea*. Known to the Romans as Autumnal Fever, this malady was seasonal, striking in the summer and fall and had a remittent or relapsing nature. It was sometimes accompanied by "dropsy," the swelling of the joints. It has been proposed that Richard suffered from tick-borne relapsing fever (Salleres, 2002, p.258). It was endemic in the Middle East at the time. He was sick for over three months.

At that point, Richard abandoned his plan to capture Jerusalem because of his poor health and treated for peace with Saladin, the Muslim leader. An eyewitness wrote "as his illness became very grave, the King despaired of recovering his health. Because of this he was much afraid, both for the others as well as for himself. Among the many things which did not pass unnoticed by his wise attention, he chose, as the least inconvenient course, to seek to make a truce rather than to desert the depopulated land altogether and to leave the business unfinished as all the others had done who left the groups in the ships. The king was puzzled and unaware of anything better that he could do." Richard returned to

Haifa seeking medical treatment (Addison, 1842).

He left the Holy Land in October of 1192, and went back to Europe only to resume fighting again with the French. He died in Châlus, near Limoges in central France, on April 6, 1199. He had been wounded in the left shoulder while fighting without wearing chain mail for protection. His cause of death was probably gangrene and/or septicemia from the infected wound. His embalmed heart has been exhumed and studied, but not subjected to DNA analysis due to degradation. Any bacteria that were found associated with it were assumed to be post mortem attachments (Charlier, et al. 2013).

The mass migration in sequential waves of tens of thousands of Crusaders from Europe to the Eastern Mediterranean led many of them directly through tick risky forests and forest edges. For thousands of crusaders this journey was a major challenge. Fevers and epidemics were often mentioned by those recounting life in army encampments along the way. While we will never know exactly which infections occurred, tick-borne infections including *Borrelia* were present in Europe at the time.

Scurvy is the nutritional deficiency that results from insufficient dietary intake of Vitamin C. While the loss of teeth is perhaps the best-known consequence in severe cases, an individual may die from spontaneous bleeding if scurvy continues for a long enough time. It is clearly described in the troops during a number of Frankish Crusader sieges. In the case of King Richard, his access to raw honey may have ameliorated the risk of scurvy. Raw honey is a source of between 2.5 (Hayak,1942) and 52 mg. of Vitamin C per tablespoon (Chua L. et al, 2013). The pupura rash of land scurvy, however, may have sometimes been confused with the rashes of Lyme disease or relapsing fever.

In a Crusader army it must have been very difficult to maintain personal hygiene, eat an adequate diet or live a lifestyle that would have lessoned the risk of contracting any one of the wide range of diseases that existed. In consequence, thousands appear to have died from various diseases in the Latin East. Lyme disease and co-infections need to be included on the list. (Phillips, 2017).

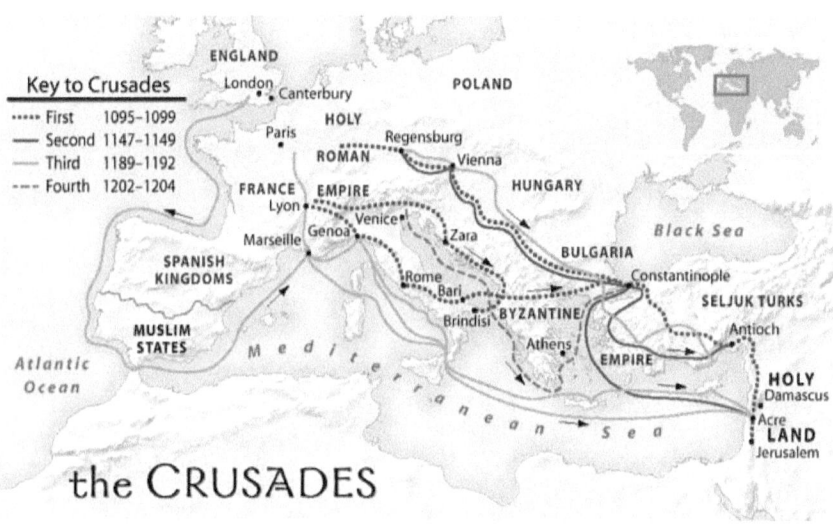

Figure 44. Some Crusader routes through Europe wound through tick-risky forested areas, including near the places where Ötzi lived his life. www.islamproject.org.

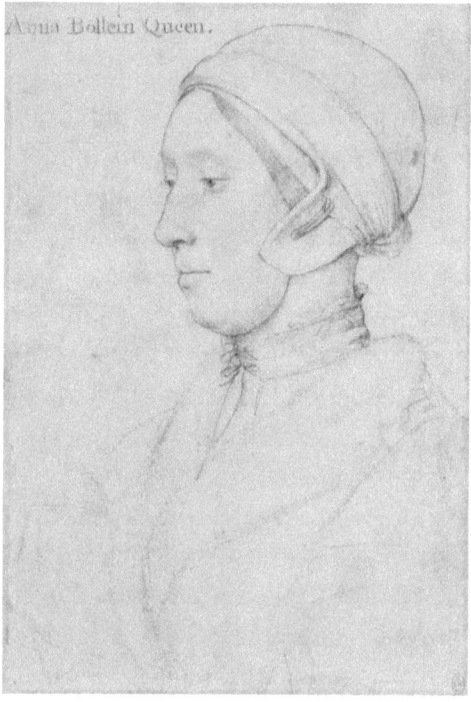

Figure 45. Drawing of Anne Boleyn, showing a 'wen' or swollen gland on her jaw, by Hans Holbein the younger, before 1536. British Library.

WHEN LYME DISEASE SWEAT: BABESIA

In March of 2012, the Health Protection Agency of the United Kingdom issued a warning to those who planned on interacting with the English and Welsh countryside that spring "to beware of ticks that carry Lyme disease." Experts estimated that between 2,000 and 3,000 infections would occur in England and Wales that year, and most of which would go unrecorded (The Daily Mail, March 28, 2012). Warning signs about Lyme disease were posted near Mortimer Forest, the modern remnant of what had been an ancient Saxon hunting forest located on the border between Wales and the English West Midlands, near the town of Ludlow (www.forestry.gov.uk). By 2017, warning signs had been added at Windsor Great Park(Occor, May 18,2017) and Lord Astor of

Hever was making a speech about the spread of Lyme disease at the House of Lords in London (www.youtube/watch?v=-FbmcEsK5YQ&feature=youtube).

In England in 1502, however, Mortimer Forest would have had no posted Lyme disease warning signs. The forest, along with the deer that inhabited it, were owned by the nobility and used for recreational hunting by the upper classes. Ludlow was an important Tudor stronghold during the rule of King Henry VII. One of the first acts of his parliament in 1485 had made unauthorized night hunting in private forests a felony punishable with death. The Tudors took their rights to hunt in their forests seriously (Bergenroth, G.A. Ed.,1862).

In the spring of 1502 the king sent his newlywed heir-presumptive, Prince Arthur, to Ludlow to preside over a Council of Wales and the Marches. The prince was accompanied by his teenaged blushing bride, Catherine of Aragon. Described as " a great beauty," short in stature, with long red hair, wide blue eyes, a round face, and fair complexion, she was an excellent and avid deer hunter. The young couple stayed at a hunting lodge in Ludlow and may have participated in the hunt in the nearby forest. Both Catherine and Arthur soon became ill with the then endemic *Sweating Sickness*[hereafter *The Sweat*]. Prince Arthur died on April 2, 1502. Catherine survived (Fraser,1992, p. 24 and Weir, 1991, p.15).

The Sweat was first noted as appearing in England in 1485 at the very beginning of the Tudor Dynasty. Emerging during the final campaign of the War of the Roses, it resurfaced in force in 1508 and again in 1517, resulting in a more deadly epidemic. It struck at Oxford and Cambridge and in some towns it was described as claiming half of the cities population. In 1528 the sweating sickness broke out in London and then quickly spread over the whole of England. It forced the Royal Court to break up and King Henry VIII to abandon his summer tour and flee in search of safety. That outbreak also struck across much of northern and eastern Europe. *The Sweat* falls out of the English history books after about 1551(Twaites, Taviner & Gant, 1997).

Two early physicians, Thomas Le Forestier and John Caius, are firsthand sources for almost all of the extant medical information we know about what they called a "pestilence." Le Forestier observed the first epidemic of *The Sweat* in 1485. He wrote that " this sickness cometh with a grete swetyng and stynkyng, with rednesse of the face and of all the body, and a contynual thurst, with a grete hete and hedache"(Le Forrestier, 1490).He attributed the epidemic to the soldiers of Henry Tudor, whose landing in Wales had "by so short a time preceded the first appearance of the disease." That army had been raised in the neighborhood of Rouen, France. While there is no description of any disease like *The Sweat* existing around Rouen prior to the departure of Henry Tudor for England, nearly 250 years later, a disease resembling it "in nearly every particular" made its appearance in the lower Seine, the very region where Henry's force had earlier been raised (Heyman, Simons,&Cochez, 2014).

Le Forestier noted that black marks were sometimes found on the skin of *The Sweat* victims (McSweegan, 2004), whereas John Caius, writing in 1551's *A Boke or Counseil against the Disease Commonly Called the Sweate or the Sweating Sickness*, found that no lesions appeared on the skin. The disease, he wrote, may have been seen before in association with warfare: among the Greeks at the siege of Troy where it killed dogs, horses, and humans, during Emperor Octavius' attacks on Cantabria in North Western Spain, and among the the Turks at Rhodes. Caius associated it with the weather. It was more likely to occur "if winter be hot & drie, somer hot and moist (a fit time for sweates), the spring colde and drye, the fall hot & moist." The final epidemic struck in 1551 during the reign of King Edward VI. It began at Shrewsbury in the middle of April, proceeded to "Ludlow, Prestene, and other places in Wales, then to Westchester, Coventry, Oxford, and other towns in the South, and such as were in and about the ways to London." This epidemic became "notable on the seventh of July, had diminished by August, and ceased altogether in September." Caius wrote that "we see this sweating sickness …..to be oft in England, but never entreth Scotland (except the borders)." The symptoms of the disease followed a specific

course. It started very suddenly with flu-like symptoms, a sense of apprehension, headaches, cold shivers, muscle aches and fatigue. This was followed by abdominal pain and vomiting then a hot and sweating stage that was accompanied by headaches and delirium. The patient would also suffer chest pains and encounter difficulty breathing-feeling a 'marvelous heaviness' and a strong desire to sleep. Death usually occurred within 24 hours (Caius, 1551).

Patients who remained alive for a longer period of time usually survived the affliction but were given no immunity against subsequent attacks. Cardinal Wolsey is recorded as being repeatedly afflicted. Anne Boleyn wrote him in 1528 to say that "touching your grace's trouble with the sweat, I thank our Lord that them I desired and prayed for are escaped"(Cheregato,1882).

The question of whether the disease was a vector borne disease or transmitted person to person is a matter of debate. *The Sweat* does seem to have spread along roads and communication routes traveled by people and herds of animals. But person to person transmission is usually facilitated by close contact during the winter season. Influenza, for example, reaches a peak in late December and early January in the modern United Kingdom (Public Health England, Winter 2013/14). All accounts agree on the summer preponderance for the sweating sickness. All five epidemics disappeared with the onset of winter.

Drs. Caius and Le Forestier believed that the disease for the most part targeted soldiers and upper class men of status falling "chiefly or rather upon men, and those of the best age as between thirty and forty years. Few women, nor children, nor old men died thereof"Caius). A study of parish death records found that while it varied from village to village, the male preponderance observed by Cauis holds true for London, but in other areas it hit a more varied demographic, included women and that there were often multiple mortalities within families and social groupings that shared a habitat(Dyer, 1997). Although affecting towns, *The Sweat* was largely a rural phenomena with limited demographic impact and some endemic characteristics(Hunter,1991).

The Sweat did made an indelible mark in English history by eliminating Prince Arthur from the line of succession and infecting two [and possibly a third] of the wives of Henry VIII. Arthur's widow Catherine of Aragon survived *The Sweat* and went on to marry Henry as her second husband. Anne Boleyn married the king after he divorced Catherine for failing to produce a male heir. Anne herself lost her head when she too failed to produce a son. Both Catherine and Anne had probably received the finest of medical care while battling *The Sweat*.

What treatment did they receive from their attending physicians? Cauis gives us some clues. The disease was thought to be caused by "evil mists and exhalations drawn out of the ground by the sun in the heat of the year," so many recommended treatments attempted to ameliorate the air. Cauis described a series of vinegar based tinctures to perfume the room of the afflicted. He states that "cleanliness is a great help to health, my advise is that all your clothes be sweet smelling and clean, and that you wash your hands and face not in warm water, but with rose water and vinegar rosate[a vinegar made with rose petals] cold, or else with the fair water and vinegar wherein the piles or barks of oranges and pomegranates are sodden...for so you shall close the pores against the air, that it readily enters not, and cool and temper those parts so washed, according to the right intent in curing this disease."

When going outside Cauis suggested repellents-to " have in your hande either an handkerchief with vinegar and rose water, or a little musk balle of nutmegs, maces, cloves, saffron, and cinnamon." Herbal treatments included the strewing of wild tansy, rue, and mogwort [note: wormwood or artemisia, is still used to treat malaria](White, 1997) or feverfew [note: also known as bachelor's buttons, also found on a Neanderthal grave, is an anti-inflammatory used to treat migraine headaches and arthritis] (wedmd.com) could be administered. Cauis recommended the daily use "of the syrups of Pomegranates, Lemons, and Sorell[note:all are excellent sources of Vitamin C]…juniper berries...and in the mouth a piece of …. the root of *enula campana* [a powerful antiseptic and bactericide] steeped in vinegar rosate"(Caius, 1551).

Both Le Forestier and Caius recommended landscape modifications to avoid infection. Both suggested that dead carcasses should be buried, especially "deadde menne in Warres" that were left "rotting above the ground" [Dr. Le Forestier ended up spending three years in the Tower of London for critiquing the clean up after the Battle at Bosworth Field](LeForrestier,1490). Ditches should be dammed and mud and puddles of stagnant water cleaned up and "in drying the moist with fires, either in houses or chambers, or on that side of the cities, town, and houses that lieth toward the infection and wind coming together, chiefly in mornings and evenings, either by burning the stubble in the field or windfallings in the woods." Caius stated "of like policy for purging the air were the bonfires made (as I suppose) for a long time hetherto used in the middle of summer, not only for vigils [probably referred to the traditional practice of leaping over these bonfires, and of driving cattle through them]." He advised people to eat well and get enough exercise so that they would be healthy to fight off infections. Finally, he advised prayer. "If other causes there be supernatural, them I leave to the divines to search, and the diseases thereof to cure, as a matter with out the compasse of my faculties" (Caius,1551).

Catherine of Aragon survived her bout with *The Sweat*. She was probably held in quarantine after her sickness for a month, a standard post-plague method used for disease control. She then spent eight years in limbo, kept in England when King Henry VII refused to allow her to return to her family in Spain. Catherine may be one of the earliest and well documented victims of chronic Lyme disease in history. She was periodically in ill health for the rest of her life.

In the summer of 1504 Catherine was taken ill with a mystery illness which kept her confined to bed with fatigue. She was subject to fits of fever and shivering and at times it was feared that she would die. In 1505 she was again confined to bed, suffering from "tertian fevers" throughout November and December. Even the Pope was concerned about her health, writing that "Catherine does not have the full power of her own body." He worried that ...devotions and fasting" would "stand in the way of

her physical health and the procreation of children..." Her own doctor stated that she suffered one continuous bout of illness that lasted for six years after her arrival in "unhealthy" England. The symptoms were varied and erratic.

They included 'derangement of the stomach,' hot sweats, cold sweats, fevers that came every other day, summer colds and summer coughs that baffled the physicians. She would complain, on the same day of 'suffering cold and heat.' A worried Spanish ambassador wrote that "she does not menstruate well." Another observer wrote that, "the only pains of which she now suffers are moral afflictions beyond the knowledge and ability of her physician.' Modern researchers, not surprisingly, have piled on by delegating her ailments to the realm of the psychological [it was all in her head!]. One even suggesting the she just needed love (Tremlett, 2010).

Love did come but it did not cure her afflictions. Indeed, it may have made them worse because she was expected to produce a male heir. Catherine married Henry VIII in 1509, after she had received a special dispensation from the Pope to marry her dead husband's brother. Between 1510 and 1518, Catherine became pregnant six times. On January 31,1510, she gave birth to a stillborn daughter. Her confessor, Fray Diego, reported that it was"without any other pain except that one knee pained her the night before." For several months after the labour, her abdomen remained rounded and even seemed to grow bigger, a symptom of a possible infection. In 1511, she gave birth to a boy named Henry who only lived for two months. In 1513, she gave birth to a stillborn son, and then gave birth to another boy who died within hours in 1515. Finally, Catherine bore a healthy daughter in 1516, who would later became Queen Mary I. It took two years for her to conceive again with a pregnancy that ended in another short-lived daughter (Fraser, and Bergenroth, Ed.,1868).

When, in 1528, the dreaded *Sweat* hit the English Royal Court again, it scared Henry VIII, who had seen his wife and sister sickened with a chronic condition and lost his only brother to the disease. It may have made him even more aware that he had no male heir. By then, Henry's attentions had begun to turn towards

Anne Boleyn.

On June 16,1528, one of Anne's ladies in waiting fell ill with *The Sweat*. Henry VIII and the court quickly fled London, seeking refuge from the epidemic. Anne Boleyn was moved to her family home at Hever Castle in Kent. The King, accompanied by Queen Catherine, 'began a most meticulous round of religious observances'(Ives, 2004, 100).This did not stop Henry from writing to his beloved Anne. He wrote that he 'would gladly bear half of your illness to make you well.' He also wrote to reassure her that 'few women or none have this malady.' Anne's father, Thomas Boleyn soon became ill. William Carey, Anne's brother-in-law, succumbed to the disease.

The king sent his second-best doctor, William Butts, because 'the physician in whom I put most trust is now at this time absent when he could most do me pleasure.' Henry urged Anne to 'to be guided by Butts' advice in your illness' so that they might be together again soon (Henry VIII, p.22). Anne and her father recovered. Within about a month, after an imposed period of quarantine, Anne was back at court. Anne Boleyn survived her experience with *The Sweat* and eventually became Henry VIII's wife (Ives,2004, 101).

Anne was married to Henry VIII for less than four years. During that time, she also had difficulty carrying a child to a full term. She gave birth to their daughter who became Queen Elizabeth I in 1533. Subsequently, she miscarried two or three times, including a three and a half month fetus which "seemed to be a male child,"according to Ambassador Chapuys. He commented, "she has miscarried of her savior." Anne was executed in 1536 (Chapuys,dispatch to Charles V dated February 10, 1536).

After her execution, the king had ordered all likenesses of Anne to be destroyed. Contemporary descriptions of Anne, moreover, were rarely objective and were influenced by the religious, political and cultural mores of her times: viewing her either as a paradigm of religious virtue or as a witch (Ives, 2004). Ann is described as having dark auburn hair and dark eyes, olive skin. She had a "wen" on her neck and possibly a tiny extra nail on the little finger of her right hand or what is described as having a

witch mark on her neck and six fingers on her left hand (Wyatt, G. 1968). The only extant drawing of Anne by Holbein appears to show her with a badly swollen gland below her jaw [see page 165]

Various theories have been proposed as to the origins of *The Sweat*. It has been proposed that the clinical manifestations of *The Sweat* are similar to hantavirus pulmonary syndrome (hereafter HPS). A critique of this theory is that HPS is only found in the Americas, not Europe, whereas in Eurasia, the hantaviruses produce a hemorrhagic fever with renal syndrome. Imagining *The Sweat* as a New World hantavirus that was transported back to England, is critiqued as meaning that the first outbreak would have had to take place after 1492 not in 1485 (Heyman, 2014). Some historians have also proposed an earlier date for the establishment of the English contact with the New World through the fishery and on-shore cod drying operations(Fagan, 2006). HPS, however, does not involve extreme sweating.

Another critique of the HPS hypothesis involves the debate over whether *The Sweat* was transmitted from human to human, as hantaviruses are not usually spread in this way. *The Sweat i*s described as following human communication routes which suggests person to person contagion. However, the spread might also represent a simultaneous clustering of infected tick, mouse, and migrating bird populations. Exposure may have progressed through exposure to peri-domestic ticks. It is possible that a novel virus with sweating symptoms evolved , afflicted, and then declined in Medieval England. Regarding vectors of a potential hantavirus, mouse numbers increase during the summer and spike periodically as a consequence of mast years, when seed producing trees like oaks produce particularly prodigious amount of food. "It probably only needed certain circumstances to provoke repeated large-scale outbreaks" of tick-borne disease (Ostfeld, et al, 2006).

The microbiologist Edward McSweegan [the blogger known as Relative Risk] has proposed that *The English Sweating Sickness* was caused by the inhalation of *Bacillus anthracis* [anthrax] caused by the willy nilly dispersal of raw wool throughout the English countryside between 1485 and 1551. He found that the symptoms that occurred during the attacks with weaponized

anthrax after 9/11/2001 included copious sweating, exhaustion, sudden onset and in five cases, agonizing deaths. Patients required mechanical ventilation and antibiotics (McSweegan, 2004). Although this attempt to normalize anthrax poisoning is compelling, the wool trade was in a diminished condition in 1485, at the time of the initial outbreak of *The Sweat* and during The War of the Roses.

The Merchant Adventurers were indeed beginning to exert control on the London-Antwerp wool cloth trade at that time, but they were not chartered as a legal monopoly until 1496 and England did not negotiate The *Intercursus Magnus* until 1506. By 1551, landholders had indeed begun increasing the size of their flocks which by the seventeenth century would find ruminants outnumbering humans by three to one in the cleared pastures of the English rural landscape.

As a historian, it is difficult to suspend all knowledge about this time period to subscribe to this theory for the cause of *The Sweat*. While this article does not propose that anyone was mailing envelopes full of weaponized anthrax spores around the Royal Court, everyone, including elites like Mary Tudor, Anne Boleyn, Prince Arthur, Cardinal Wolsey, Catherine of Aragon and most of the Royal Privy Council were unlikely to have been wallowing around in raw wool, sheep droppings, and anthrax spores (Redstone, 1902). All of these people, however, as well as Sweat survivors Thomas Boleyn and William Carey, participated in one of the most popular and tick-risky of Tudor elite pastimes: The Hunt.

The hypothesis of this study is that *The Sweat* was a tick borne set of co-infections. Lyme disease is the result of an infection based on a persistent spiral: *Borrelia*. A description of tick attachment occurring on an island off the coast of Scotland can be found from 1764 (Summerton, N. 1995) and studies of DNA taken from ticks in the British Natural History Museum collection show that *Borrelia* were present in England during Victorian times (Hubbard et al., 1998). It has plagued Europeans for at least 5300 years (Hall, S., November 2011).

The symptoms of *The Sweat* can be explained by applying knowledge from modern Lyme disease research studies to the history. Humans are infected when they become incidental blood meal hosts after interacting with tick habitat, usually at forest edges. The *Ixodes* life cycle is dependent on the leaf litter of England's oak filled forests for protection in winter. Although ticks can become active anytime the ambient temperature rises above freezing, Lyme disease is predominantly a summer affliction.

Some years, ticks are more abundant than in others (Ostfield & Schauber, 2001). This is an ageless phenomena. Writing in the early seventeenth century, John Josselyn noted that "there be infinite numbers of tikes hanging upon the bushes in summer time that will cleave to man's garments and creep into his breeches eating themselves in a short time into the very flesh of a man. I have seen the stockins of those that have gone through the woods covered with them"(Josselyn, 1663).

It is also a modern experience. A recent three day hike in Western Canada, for example, resulted in a good description of what the experience of interacting with a tick infested area two years after a mast year and immediately following a warm winter is like. The newspaper headline reads "Tick-mageddon!" A total of over four hundred ticks were removed from the clothing of one intrepid outdoors woman. "The ticks buried themselves inside pant legs, down under shirt collars, and behind ears." She stated that on all her backcountry trips, she had never seen ticks that bad. "We were just overwhelmed. We were taking them off as much as we could," she said. "After we washed in the evening and put clean clothes on, still they were on us." Days after returning home, she's still battling ticks, she's still finding them in her home on piles of laundry and even in a cupboard. "They're hard to get rid of, you'll check yourself and then you'll look again thirty seconds later and there's one on your stomach again. I don't understand where they come from!" She is well aware that ticks carry Lyme disease and will be on the lookout for any indication of infection (Glowaski, L. May 19,2017).

Ixodes borne relapsing fever *[Borrelia miyamotoi]*brings reoccurring high fevers with multiple febrile episodes. Some

patients develop gastrointestinal problems[vomiting, nausea, diarrhea], cardiac and respiratory symptoms, including shortness of breath, and neurological symptoms like dizziness and confusion(www.medscape.com, June 12, 2015). *Ixodes* ticks in North America have been found presently to carry the co-infection *Powassan Virus*, which can have a thirty percent fatality rate (www.cdc) In a modern study of over three thousand patients with chronic Lyme disease, it was found that over fifty percent also had co-infections, with thirty percent reporting two or more co-infections. The most common co-infection is *Babesia*. The hallmark of *Babesia* is **drenching sweats** (Johnson, et al., 2014).

Babesia starts with high fever and chills. It's psychological manifestations include anxiety and panic attacks. As the infection progresses, patients can develop fatigue, headache, muscle aches, chest pain, hip pain, and shortness of breath ("air hunger"). Complications of severe *Babesia* infection have been found to be acute respiratory failure, disseminated intravascular coagulation, and congestive heart and renal failure. In one review of patients admitted to a single hospital, three out of thirty four patients treated for *Babesia* died. In another study, sixty six percent of patients with Lyme disease also had *Babesia* and fifty four percent of people with *Babesia* also have Lyme disease. When Lyme is acquired with a co-infection, symptoms can be more severe and last longer. Both Lyme and *Babesia* can become chronic afflictions (Krause, P.J. et al.1994). *Babesia* has also been found to have been transferred in utero from mother to child (Feder, et al., 2014, Saetre, et al 2017).

Chronic Lyme Disease is a multi-system illness that has diverse musculoskeletal, neuropsychiatric and/or cardiovascular manifestations that result from ongoing infection with pathogenic members of the *Borrelia* spirochete complex often associated with other tick-borne pathogens. Patients have Lyme compatible symptoms and signs that are either consistently or variably present for six or more months. When applied to the past, it is assumed that the patients were not administered antibiotics, although many traditional herbal remedies have antibiotic qualities.

One modern victim described his experience with Chronic

Lyme Disease. "I got the classic Lyme disease for each successive summer, for five years, every August, like this black lung, flu-like symptoms, sweating to death in my bed...The first time was the worst of all...And I really thought this is it, I'm not going to live. I was lying in bed saying, 'I'm going to die of Lyme disease" (Young, May 22,2017).

The relationship between Lyme disease and its co-infections to fertility and pregnancy outcomes has been studied. Anecdotal evidence suggests that Lyme can cause irregular menstrual cycles and sometimes a complete cessation of periods(Horowitz, 2013). The CDC website states that Lyme disease acquired during pregnancy may lead to infection of the placenta and possible stillbirth (www.cdc.gov). One study, which compared live births in an endemic area to those in a non-endemic area found no statistical difference in outcomes other that a slight increase in polydactylism and hemangioma in the endemic area [Interestingly, two attributes sometimes attributed to Anne Boleyn] that could be explained by non-Lyme related variables (Schlesinger, P.A et al.,1985).

However, pregnancy outcomes with the congenital anomalies associated with miscarriages, still-births, or perinatal infant deaths were excluded by that study's design(Williams, et al.1995).When these outcomes are included, Lyme disease has been found to be associated with birth defects, fetal death in utero, fetal death at term, and infant death after birth (MacDonald, 1989). Birth defects included congenital heart disease during the first week of life. Histologic examination of autopsy material has found *Borrelia* spirochetes in the placenta, spleen, fetal myocardium, kidneys, liver, arachnoid space of fetal mid brain, and bone marrow (Schlesinger, 1985).

One full term infant, used as a case study, was born with multiple anomalies including hydrocephalus, omphalocoele, clubfoot, spina bifida, and meningomyelocoele. After developing respiratory distress, the infant died four hours after birth. Autopsy disclosed a large ventriculoseptal defect as an additional malformation. Spirochetes were identified by immuno-histo chemistry in a retrospective examination of fetal tissue (MacDonald,1989).

One mother had a history of suffering from two miscarriages that were never examined histologically. Her third pregnancy resulted in a male fetus that was aborted in the emergency room. Its autopsy disclosed no external or internal anomalies. Culture yielded *Borrelia burgdorferi* and other bacteria from the fetal kidney tissue (Lavoe, et al, 1987).

Another case study of a full term male infant who developed respiratory distress in the first hour of life and died twenty-three and one half hours later revealed otherwise normal appearing placental villi which contained *Borrelia burgdorferi* spirochetes (MacDonald 1989). In a case study of 102 children born to mothers who were either untreated or partially treated for lyme, sixty six percent reported a difficult pregnancy. In mothers who were being treated for active lyme, eighty five percent of the newborns were normal. In those who had not received antibiotics, only thirty three percent of neonates were born normal(Weber,et al, 1988). Gestational Lyme borreliosis has been described in 5 of 19 pregnancies (26%) resulting in "syndactyly, cortical blindness, intrauterine fetal death, prematurity, and rash"(Markowitz, 1986).

Other co-infections also cause reproductive problems. *Bartonella* has been found to be passed to the unborn, causing chronic infections and birth defects. In one study a 10-year-old boy was chronically ill from birth. His sibling died due to a heart defect at nine days of age. Microbiological tests indicated that the mother [and father] had been exposed to *Bartonella*. The same bacteria was found in both children, one shortly after birth and the other ten years later, indicating that they may have become infected while in utero (Breitschwerdt, et al, 2010). Studies from rural East Africa have shown an increased incidence of spontaneous abortion, low neonatal birth weight, and preterm labour among pregnant women with tick-borne relapsing fever (Hussein, et al 1997). Lyme and/or co-infections have also been found to cause miscarriages in horses(Johnson, R.,2009), cattle(February,1987) and dogs (University of Bristol, January 25, 2012).

The fertility problems of Catherine of Aragon and Anne Boleyn are the stuff of legends, well supported by primary source

references. There were commonalities between the two women, aside from a marriage partner, both having suffered and survived the English sweating sickness, as even Henry VIII wrote, a rare occurrence. They inhabited the same landscape of the English Royal Court and both were fond of the hunt, often accompanying Henry VIII on his forays into the Royal Forest in quest of deer(Kinney & Swain, 2000). Both suffered through repeated miscarriages and stillbirths. Did Catherine of Aragon and Anne Boleyn contract Lyme disease and/or the co-infection *Babesia* ? History reveals that:

1. Although Lyme disease is usually considered to be a new affliction that was discovered in 1975, with the B*orrelia's* spirals being first discovered within a tick in 1982, it is in reality an extremely old bacteria. The fossilized remains of its twenty-five million year old ancestors have been found preserved within amber, as have some of the co-infections(Poinar, 2014). We also now know that an infected human walked the earth over five thousand years ago (Hall, S., November 2011).

2. There is a Tale of Two Lymes raging in the modern medical community (Frisch, T. 2010). Lyme disease is considered by a large faction of the medical community to be little more than a nuisance illness. Treat it with a few weeks of antibiotics and it all goes away. In contrast, Lyme disease can viewed as a chronic, potentially deadly disease that progresses into various organ systems. Lyme disease can be viewed as complex, difficult to treat, hard to cure, life altering affliction that can continue to cause chronic problems after the initial acute infection. This study, due to personal experience, supports the second stance and the idea that it has played an important role in shaping history.

3. England was in the middle of The War of the Roses for over thirty years beginning in 1455 and ending on the Field at Bosworth in 1485, the place where *The Sweat* first broke out in England. The war created environmental disturbance. Manpower was sent into

various armies, fields went untended, leaves were not burned off, which resulted in re-forestation in some areas.

4. The war was finally won by Henry Tudor. He arrived from exile in France in 1485 with an army consisting of thirty shiploads of soldiers, horses, and supplies that had been raised in the Rouen area of Normandy. Henry's army would be augmented by Welsh supporters as he marched between the August 7 landing site on the Welsh seacoast and Bosworth. Henry had to march around collecting volunteers along the way. The army camped along the way, often in forest edge environments. It is possible that 1483 or 1484 had been a mast year for the oak trees of the central section of England and that the prior winter had been warm so that ticks and mice had been well fed and more likely to survive. These mice and migrating birds would have already been infected with *Borrelia, Babesia* and other co-infections which had been passed along when *Ixodes* tick nymphs had taken a blood meal in the spring. The nymphs then grew up to be an over abundance of infected adult ticks by August.

5. They quested in forest edges. As opportunistic questers, ticks jump on to whatever blood meal host presents itself. What they got in 1485 was an army of three thousand men accompanied by horses and associated dogs. By the time they reached the field at Bosworth fifteen days later on August 22, soldiers were beginning to be afflicted by *The Sweat* (Hutton, 1813).

6. After the death of King Richard III, whose crown was hidden in a hawthorn bush before being placed on Henry Tudor's head, as he stood under an oak tree. King Henry VII then started a march towards London arriving either on August 28 or September 7. He left behind environmental devastation: a field full of unburied dead bodies and a stream so tinged with the blood of the slain that for a long time the residents could not drink from it. Thomas Le Forestier, the chronicler of the first outbreak of what he called the *Dread Sweat* ended up locked in the Tower of London for three

years because he noted the health concerns that may have been created by those rotting cadavers (Le Forestier, 1490).

6. No outbreak of *The Sweat* was noted beforehand at the point of departure for Henry's army from France. The outbreak is associated with the legendary March through Wales, the Stanley forces at Bosworth, and the subsequent 7 or 17 day long march to London by a group of men who had extensive interactions with a forest edge environment along the way (Heyman,et al.2014).

7. Subsequently, there were periodic outbreaks of The Sweat with a final epidemic noted in 1551.

8.*The Sweat* was a rural affliction, often afflicting groups of people[especially men] or families who shared an environment. In London, the victims were almost exclusively male although in parish records, there is a more even balance of afflicted more endemic in nature. *The Sweat* of 1551 afflicted different areas differently, with death rates varying from 1.2 % to upwards of 10 % of the population (Taviner,et al., 1998).

9. It was a summer affliction.

10.The affliction did not create immunity. Arthur Tudor may have had fallen sick in November 1501 only to succumb the next Spring to a second attack. Cardinal Wolsey was afflicted several times. Noted people, who were more likely to make the historic records, who suffered from *The Sweat* sometimes remained chronically ill afterwards. Mary Tudor exhibited signs of failing health after her bout with the sweating sickness in 1518 and was chronically ill until she died in 1533.The most chronicled post Sweat victim who remained ill afterwards was Catherine of Aragon(Derbyshire, May 20, 2002).Lyme disease does not afford immunity for subsequent attacks and often becomes a chronic affliction.

11. These symptoms described by Le Forrestier and John Caius can be explained as an epidemic of a particular virulent form of Lyme disease that was amplified by the co-infection *Babesia* and a tick-borne virus.

12. The recommendation of Dr. John Caius, who treated patients with *The Sweat,* include landscape modifications like the burning off of fields and forest understory, insect repellants like vinegar, rue, and tansy, and herbal remedies known to be effective for *Borrelia* and *Babesia* infections in modern times, especially enula root and wormwood (artemesia).

13. During the span of the Tudor monarchs, England underwent population growth and rapid and massive de-forestation. Trees in Tudor England were heavily coppiced. An economic turn toward not only wool production but cloth making, especially after the post 1572 St. Bartholomew's Day mass migration of Huguenot weavers into England, filled newly opened fields with sheep which can be effective tick mops (Porter, et al. May 20, 2010).

14. The propensity of *The Sweat* towards mid-aged male and upper class victims can be explained by a greater amount of interactions with forest edges. Hunting was an exclusionary activity retained by the nobility and upper class, with mostly male participants. Hunting Laws declared that was a sport for "Kings and Princes, and therefore not to be used by every common Person, but only by such of the Nobility and others who have Authority from the King, or from his Justice in Eyre, or other Officers of the Forest, or by such who have some good and lawful Authority so to do, and no other may hunt there." Hunting was viewed as "an essential mark of a gentleman and...was valued as a test of courage, strength, and agility..."(Kinney & Swain, 2000) It was a main"pastyme" of Henry VIII. Hunting was "a royal and aristocratic sport, almost as prestigious as warfare, and required the same courage and skills as were needed in battle. The quarry, which was usually deer, was either shot with bows and arrows, tracked down by dogs, or driven into nets," then ceremoniously killed. The deer or wild boar were chased by the King and his company on horseback. Hunting was not always a man's sport. Many times, the Queen would

accompany the King. All three of Henry's early wives spent time hunting with him. His daughter, Queen Elizabeth I, also enjoyed The Hunt (License,2016).

15. Both Anne Boleyn and Catherine of Aragon were avid hunters [as was Queen Jane Seymour, whose sole documentary record that has been preserved is an order to a park keeper "to deliver to her well-beloved the gentlemen of her sovereign lord the king's chapel-royal, two bucks of high season"(Strickland,1868, p.279).

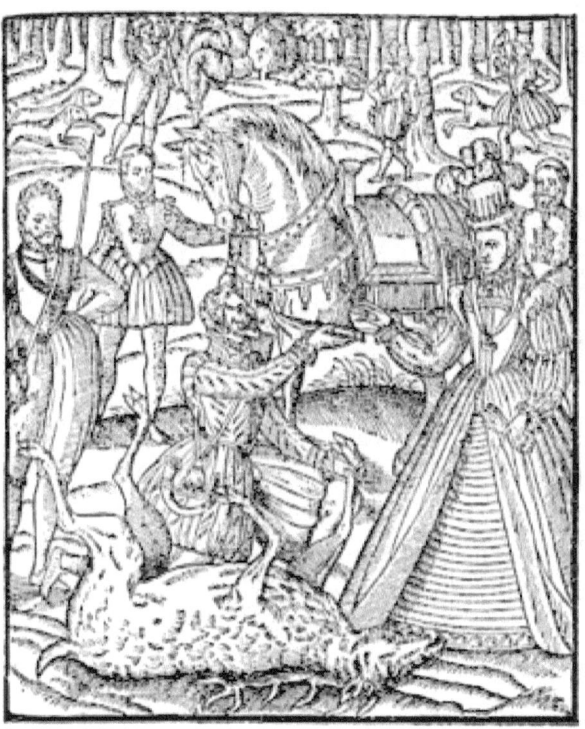

Figure 46. Hunting traditions brought elite hunters into close contact with deer. In this woodcut Queen Elizabeth is preparing to slit the throat of a deer. George Turbervile, *The Book of Hunting*, woodcut, 1576.

16. Catherine of Aragon and Anne Boleyn were both afflicted with and survived *The Sweat*.

17. Catherine of Aragon suffered for years afterwards with joint pain, unexplained and erratic illness, and was often bed ridden. Catherine had an irregular menstrual cycles and sometimes a complete cessation of her periods.

18. Both Catherine and Anne Boleyn may have suffered from chronic Lyme disease which should be considered as a possible cause for their reproductive problems. Anne Boleyn was buried without any autopsy but at death, Catherine's chest cavity was examined by the local chandler [candlemaker] while preparing her body for burial in a wax coated shroud. He reported that all of her organs appeared healthy apart from her heart, "which was quit black and hideous to look at" with a black spot attached to it. (Lehman, 2011). The disseminated intravascular coagulation associated with *Babesia* can cause both internal bleeding and clots and can give the heart a black appearance. Because red blood cells are destroyed, severe *Babesia* infection can mimic cancer. Enlarged red blood cells, swollen with the piroplasms, can impede passage through capillaries. *Babesia* also increases clotting. In worse case scenario, this can cause mini-strokes. Blockage of small blood vessels from swollen blood vessels and increased clotting are one of the main ways *Babesia* causes harm (Shaller & Mounty 2012). Some of the people who survived the most acute phase of the infection suffered from a chronic illness afterwards and lived with a diminished quality of life. Lyme disease and tick-borne co-infections are very old afflictions that remain endemic in England and other parts of the world to this very day. Lyme disease and the co-infection *Babesia* made England sweat between 1485 and 1551.

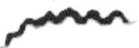

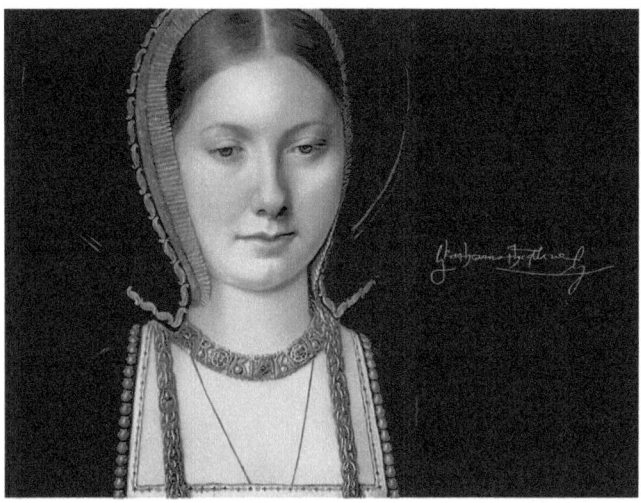

Figure 47. Portrait of a teenaged Catherine of Aragon by Michael Sittow, circa 1500-1505, painted at around the age that she contracted *The Sweat*.

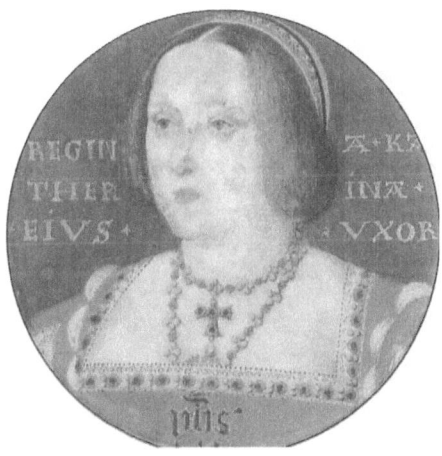

Figure 48. Miniature Portrait of Catherine of Aragon by Lucas Horenbout, circa 1528. By her early 40's Catherine was post menopausal, had suffered from chronic illness for over twenty-five years, had been pregnant six times but had only one surviving child, and was about to enter messy divorce proceedings.

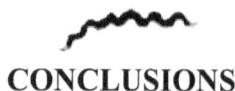

CONCLUSIONS

"People should not be blind to the possibility that things that are hailed as new may well be what has always been here."

Vanya Gant, St. Thomas' Hospital, London, U.K.

"As long as humans have been around, I'm sure that they suffered from ailments caused by spirochetes carried by ticks."

Dr. George Poinar, Jr., Oregon State University.

Lyme disease and some co-infections are OLD pathogens. Lyme disease is an ancient, insidious, and ubiquitous affliction that humans have been coping with throughout history and prehistory. The ancestors of *Borrelia, Rickettsia,* and *Babesia* have been found in ticks embedded in amber that is millions of years old, showing that both these pathogens and the ticks that vector them have been on earth longer that humans have been human. Genetic studies have found that the *Borrelia burdorferi* in North America has a signature of ancient demographic processes, including spatial expansions that occurred at least on the order of thousands of years ago.

The pathogen has always been around but what has changed over time is how and where people were living and how much they were interacting with tick-risky environments. Archaic humans, like the Neanderthal and Denisovans, were the first to populate Eurasia and wander through the temperate forests that are so beloved by *Borrelia* spirochetes and *Ixodes* ticks. This influenced their immune system development. When Early Modern Humans and Archaic Humans mated, some parts of the Archaic Human innate immune system recognition was passed on to human populations. Inherited Archaic TLRs can mount sustained attacks against *Borrelia*.

Some mammals, like deer and mice, having been a blood meal host for ticks infected with *Borrelia* for millions of years, have developed immune systems that are able to cope with this

infection. Humans have not. *Borrelia* is recognized by human Toll Like Receptor 2 [TLR2] showing 400,000 years of experience confronting this pathogen. It has gotten into our human bones for millennia. Neanderthals and the Early Modern Human Hunter-Gatherers that followed them in time into the tick-risky forests suffered from high levels of bone infections. *Borrelia's* ability to screw its way deeply into bone marrow. When humans chopped down the forests and began to live in modified Agrarian, then Industrialized and/or Urban settings, bone infection and arthritis diminished. When they moved into the Post-Industrial suburbs of the Mid-Twentieth Century, bone infections and arthritis came back with a vengeance. This may be related to the presence of *Borrelia*.

How an individual responds to Lyme disease is related to genetics and variations in pathogen history. Some ancestral groups have had more experience with *Borrelia*, both biologically and culturally, than others. The Chinese who refuged from the Last Glacial Maxima in a temperate forested area, if Traditional Chinese medical practices are indicative, had more consistent experience with tick-borne infections than the Yamnaya of Central Asia, whose ancestors sheltered in the grassland and developed a horse and cattle centered culture on the mostly tick-less steppes. Early Native Americans lived in some very tick-risky areas during the same time period. African immune systems were confronted by a panoply of pathogens including a bit of *Borrelia* in some areas.

DNA haplotypes give us clues to where our ancestors have been and how variation in immune responses evolved. Human culture has developed ways to fight disease. By as early as the end of the Mesolithic, humans had learned to use fire to burn off undergrowth. They did this to facilitate hunting. Fire promoted open grassy areas to attract ruminants with food sources. Fire killed ticks. The introduction of agriculture changed the landscape that humans interacted with, brought new technologies as well as new groups of humans into Europe, and resulted in a sustained campaign of deforestation. The land became pastures and fields, that were again often managed with fire. Humans began to share the land with a diversity of domesticated animals, including cows,

horses, cats, and chickens. As the landscape matured over time it became less tick-risky.

When human ethnic groups began to coalesce, they shared haplotypes as well as cultural practices and environmental conditions. Bone infection became very low so that by the time period of the Middle Ages it was virtually non-existent. The Agrarian and Urban landscapes of Eurasia and the Americas seems to have been relatively safe from Lyme disease, with a few notably exceptions.

Warfare does a couple of things to a landscape. It diverts attention away from the land and leads to overgrowth and less maintenance, which can encourage ticks, especially if burn rates also diminish. Warfare also tends to disrupt society and move men into places that may be more "wild" and tick risky. This occurred during Thirty Years War in Europe, The War of the Roses in England, King Williams War in New England, The Crusades, and also during the spread of the Ming Empire in China. Another activity that brought people into contact with a tick-ricky forest was the elite's favorite pastime, especially in England, The Hunt.

Epidemics have two important effects on human history. First, they serve as biological screening tools favoring some immune responses over others. Sometimes, a mismatch is created. What worked for one pathogen mat be detrimental for another. Excessive deaths can also lead to less land maintenance, forest regrowth, and overgrowth which also leads to a tick risky environment. This happened after The Black Plague in Europe and The Great Pestilence of 1618 in New England and may have triggered many of the symptoms thought to be related to witchcraft affliction. Plague, smallpox and influenza have killed vast swaths of human populations. The last great pandemic was the Influenza epidemic that followed WWI. Technology can also effect landscapes. The plow expanded agricultural land use. The rise of mechanical industries with economic advantages caused farm abandonment. The modern suburb was created in response to the the automobile.

Many Traditional medical treatments, going back as far as the Neanderthals, have antibiotic and pain relieving properties that

would be useful in treating Lyme disease. These practices, in conflict with the modern definition of science, have fallen by the wayside, described as folkloric, old fashioned, and occasionally, dangerous. But they need to be rescued from history's trash bin because they may still have use, especially in an age of antibiotic overuse and resistance. One of the herbs prescribed for The English Sweating Sickness, for example, is still the basis for modern treatments for *Babesia*.

Chinese Acupuncture and Traditional Medicines have been used to treat a full spectrum of spirochetes illnesses for thousands of years. Many modern Lyme patients use Medical Marijuana, which we can thank our Yamnaya ancestors for bringing to Europe and China. These traditional herbal treatments stand available to augment modern treatments. Another traditional practice, a tool of humans since at least the Mesolithic Era, that had been discontinued in New England, is fire. This is an extremely effective method for reducing tick populations. Regularly burnings, done annually, have been found to significantly reduce tick populations. Fire use should be revisited. The trade off between air pollution and Lyme disease should be quantified to see if accommodations can be made to fire restrictions. This might eliminate Lyme disease risk in some areas. Lyme disease may be a geographically limited tick- borne infection, but it has certainly not been restricted to any particular period of time. It is threaded through time. Ticks and the pathogens they carry are formidable foes and have been for millions of years. Ticks may have developed their barbed mouths in order to hacksaw their way through the tough skin of the dinosaurs. Dinosaurs may have been infected with a wide range of tick-borne infections.

There are million year old stories written in amber. Fifteen million years ago, a monkey was sitting near a tree when it encountered a blood sucking tick. That monkey was already infected with the ancestor of *Babesia*. It found the tick in its fur, plucked it off, squished it, and threw it onto a pool of tree sap where it get stuck and became an inclusion in a piece of amber over time. Other stories about Lyme disease are written in human epigentics and immune reactions. Four hundred thousand years

ago, the Neanderthal immune system learned to recognize *Borrelia* infections. Some Lyme history is in bones. While walking through an Alpine forest 5000 years ago, Ötzi contracted Lyme disease which made its way into his bone marrow. Oral history, written down from Native American folkloric traditions, tells a story about connecting deer with rheumatism. Cultural practices, like the popularity of cock-fighting, helped chickens spread their *Borrelia* affliction around the world. Cats helped spread *Bartonella*. Then we encounter modern history. This is a particularly sad chapter of the story. Some of the children that were treated for "this newly discovered disease" in Lyme, Connecticut, have grown up into adults who are still plagued with ongoing health problems. An ever growing list of celebrities have begun to tell their Lyme stories. It seems that the point of Lyme disease research and practice should be centered around the concept of bulletproof testing and "care" but it is not.

The United States of America and many other parts of the world have a 'Lyme Disease Problem' that [after a personal twenty-years of affliction] is not being addressed. The only CDC-recommended tests for Lyme disease has a fifty percent failure rate. Untreated or undertreated Lyme results in Chronic Lyme Disease, a condition characterized by the development of severe, difficult-to-resolve symptoms. The history of the last few decades of Lyme affliction is a grim one.

In the 1970's, when Lyme Disease was a "new" disease, it attracted the attention of the American medical community. As recognition of the symptoms had spread by the 1990's, several major health insurers seem to have decided that treating it was becoming too expensive. This problem was ameliorated in several ways. At the Dearborn CDC Conference in 1994, several bands indicative of the difficult to treat neurological *Borreliosis* were removed from the blood test commonly used for diagnosis. A vaccine called Lymerix was patented by researchers associated with the Infectious Disease Society of America and brought to market in 1998. It was supposed to lower infection rates but it eventually had to be pulled when side effects garnered some bad publicity within the growing Lyme patient community (Dickson,

2015).

Based on the revised testing regiment, Lyme infection rates were reduced anyway. Insurance companies also paid Infectious Disease Society of America affiliated doctors – who were researching, not treating, Lyme disease and owned some of the vaccine patents – to establish guidelines in 2000 that said the disease could be cured with 28 days of antibiotics. Since then, this recommended short term treatment may have failed to properly treat up to forty percent of patients with Lyme disease, meaning that more than 100,000 Lyme disease patients each year are left untreated when the IDSA guidelines were followed. That does not even count the infected who have tested negative since 1994. It is an ever enlarging group.

In 2006 even more restrictive guidelines for treating Lyme disease were established, actually promoting the idea that "Lyme is a simple, rare illness that is easy to avoid, difficult to acquire, simple to diagnose, and easily treated and cured with 28 days of antibiotics.' Insurance companies treat the IDSA guidelines as 'de facto' law that must be followed by doctors and steadfastly refuse to cover any treatment outside the IDSA guidelines. One physician who was paid, according to a 1996 deposition, $560 an hour to review Lyme disease files for insurance companies almost always denied coverage, especially for Chronic Lyme Disease. (Landford, 2017).

Health Insurance companies also went after doctors who criticized the guidelines, putting their medical licenses at risk. As a result of speaking out, more than fifty physicians in New York, New Jersey, Connecticut, Michigan, Oregon, Rhode Island and Texas were investigated, disciplined, or had had their licenses removed between 1997 and 2000. The insurers also allegedly reported doctors who were treating Chronic Lyme Disease to state medical boards, leading many doctors to refuse to treat Lyme disease patients at all. The result is that many patients have been forced to travel long distances to find doctors willing to treat them, and pay thousands of dollars out of their pockets for care, or go without (Conner, 2017).

The CDC's preferential use of outdated and inaccurate

Infectious Disease Society of America guidelines for treating Lyme supports the narrative that Chronic Lyme does not exist. Thus, insurance companies are not required to cover ongoing treatment costs. The lack of recognition for this disease cannot continue. We NEED AN ACCURATE DIAGNOSTIC TEST for this disease. We need care. Instead, we get derision and have division. A strong lack of compassion seems to be the hallmark of much of the modern medical attitude towards Lyme disease. The afflicted are left without hope. Some have become profoundly mentally ill with neuroborreliosis. It is a matter of medical ethics.

    The Modern Hippocratic Oath includes the phrase, "I will not be ashamed to say I know not, and, I will remember that I remain a member of society, with special obligations to all my fellow human beings." This oath is derived from one of the earliest expressions of medical ethics in the western world and remains of significance today. Those who deny the severity of Lyme are wrong, and as the number of Lyme and co-infected afflicted grow, a tipping point will someday be reached. Lyme deniers will eventually be toppled by a tsunami of Lyme experiences.

    The main threat to public health that we confront in modern America is the erosion of faith in the motivations of some medical researchers and practitioners. Some have tried to use Lyme disease to gild their reputations and apply for lucrative drug patents while denying the experiences of thousands of infected people. I have great difficulty respecting any researcher who, knowing that this disease can be treated with antibiotics would participate in a study design that excludes treatment for the infected. Accurate testing, access to quality treatments, and a healthy life supported by a caring medical system is the aspiration for most Lyme Activists. Most patients just want their life back.

    I do have great respect for modern Lyme advocacy workers. I have also come to admire the victims of tick-borne disease that I could find rattling around in the records of the past. I have gained enormous respect for Catherine of Aragon, a historic figure that I knew very little about before I wrote this book, other than a bit about a divorce from Henry VIII. She clearly displayed great strength of character and dignity in the face of a chronic ailment

that stripped her of most of her children, her station in life, her wealth, her physical health, and in the end, life itself. Her life can serve as a cautionary tale for both the afflicted and naysayers of today. The victims of this disease can persist and resist. Any threat to public health comes from infected ticks not Lyme activists. Science has been diverted by some who saw this affliction as the road to riches and reputation, not as a public health puzzle to be solved. Lyme disease is not a limited tick-borne infection. It is an insidious disease that is becoming more and more ubiquitous, is difficult to diagnose, and can be almost incurable. Until this is acknowledged, we are at a moral impasse.

It needs to be acknowledged that there is no one-size-fits-all solution to Lyme disease. Why is this ? Because it is an affliction complicated by variables like co-infections, genetic traits that facilitate or hinder treatment, and varying environmental factors. It involves *Borrelia* that have a multi-million year head start in the fight. An approach that might work well for one person might cause a dangerous reaction in others. Antibiotics are not always the only answer. We may need to look back at the practices of our ancestors in order to go forward. There is a plethora of traditional treatment protocols-Medical Marijuana, Traditional Chinese Medicine, and Western Folkloric herbals are still available.

For the near future, Lyme advocates will continue to participate in public protests, find corruption and conspiracy where they exist, and continue to spur legislative efforts to protect our care and our caregivers. Supposedly respectable scientists will probably continue to call us names and ridicule our efforts. But I do believe that someday history will bring vindication. Belittle us if you must, but our life stories and the suffering we endure will one day be recognized, if only as a chapter of history filled with sad injustice

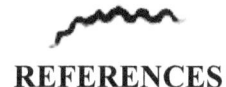

REFERENCES

Aceves-Avila, F., Medina, F, & Fraga, A. (2001, April). The antiquity of rheumatoid arthritis: a reappraisal. *J Rheumatol*, 28, 4:751-7.

Achillia, A., Olivieri, A., Soares, P., Lancionia, H., Kashanib, B.H., Perego, U., Nergadzeb, S., Carossab, V., Santagostino, M., Capomaccio,S., Felicetti, M., Al-Achkarf, W., Penedog,C., Verini-Supplizi, A., Houshmand, M., Woodward,S., Semino, O., Silvestrelli, M., Giulotto,E., Pereira, L., Bandeltj,H-J. & Torroni,A. (2012, January 30). Mitochondrial genomes from modern horses reveal the major haplogroups that underwent domestication. *PNAS,* Vol. 109, 7: 2449-2454.

Addison, C.G. (1842). *King Richard the Lionheart's experiences with the Knights Templar during the Crusades, the Journal of Geoffrey de Vinsauf who accompanied King Richard on his expedition.*

Adelson, M.E., Rao, R.V., Tilton, R.C., Cabets, K., Eskow, E., Fein, .L, Occi, J.L., Mordechai, E.(2004).Prevalence of Borrelia burgdorferi, Bartonella spp., Babesia microti, and Anaplasma phagocytophila in Ixodes scapularis ticks collected in Northern New Jersey. *J Clin Microbiology,* 42:2799-2801.

Agarwal, R. & Sze, G. (2009). Neuro-Lyme Disease: MR Imaging Findings. *Radiology,* Vol. 253, 1.

Agnetha, H., Fedor, G., Willem, T., Frans, J., van Vliet, A.J.H., van Ballegooijen, M., van der Giessen, J., Katsuhisa, T. (2012). Circumstantial evidence for an increase in the total number and activity of borrelia-infected ixodes ricinus in the Netherlands. *Parasites & Vectors,* 5: 294.

Ali, E.M., Almagboul, A.Z., Khogali, S.M., & Gergeir, U.M. (2012). Antimicrobial Activity of Cannabis sativa L. *Chinese Medicine*, 3: 61-64.

Allan, B. (2009). Influence of prescribed burns on abundance of *Amblyomma americanum* (Acari: Ixodidae) in the Missouri Ozarks. *Journal Med Entomology* 46: 1030–1036.

Allan, B., Keesing, F., Ostfeld, R. (2003). Effect of Forest Fragmentation on Lyme disease risk. *Conserv Biol* 17: 267–272.

Allen, C.S., Stephene, E.M., John, A.H., Shaun,R., Philip, W.A., Warren, A.A. (1977). Erythema Chronicum Migrans and Lyme Arthritis: The Enlarging Clinical Spectrum. *Annals of Internal Medicine*, 6: 685-698.

Allen, H., Shaver, C., Etzler, C., & Joshi, S. (2015, December 31). Autoimmune Diseases of the Innate and Adaptive Immune System including Atopic Dermatitis, Psoriasis, Chronic Arthritis, Lyme Disease, and Alzheimers Disease. *Immunochesmistry and Immunopathology.*

Allentoft,M., Sikora, M., Sjögren, K-G., Rasmussen, S., Rasmussen, M., Stenderup, J.,Damgaard, P., Schroeder,H., Ahlström,T., Vinner,L., Malaspinas, A-S., Margaryan, A., Higham,T., Chivall, D., Lynnerup,N., Harvig, L., Baron,J., Della Casa, P., Dąbrowski, P., Duffy, P., Ebel,A., Epimakhov, A., Frei, K., Furmanek,M., Gralak, T. (2015, June 11). Population genomics of Bronze Age Eurasia. *Nature* 522: 167–172.

Ammerman, A & Cavalli-Sforza, L.L.(2014).*The Neolithic Transition and the Genetics of Populations in Europe*. Princeton, N.J.: Princeton University Press.

Anan'eva ,LP, Skripnikova, IA, Barskova, VG, & Steere, AC. (1995). The clinical and serological manifestations of Lyme disease in Russia. *Ter Arkh,* 67,11:38-42.

Anderson, B. & Borns, H. (1997). *The Ice Age World: An Introduction to Quaternary History and Research.* Universitetsforlaget.

Andersen, L.W., Jacobsen, M., Vedel-Smith, C., & Jensen, T.S. (2017, July). Mice as stowaways? Colonization history of Danish striped field mice. *Biology Letters,*13: 7.

Ansari, R., Mahta, A.,Mallack, E., & Luoa, J.J. (2014, October).Hyperhomocysteinemia and Neurologic Disorders: a Review. *J Clin Neuro*logy.

Anthony, D.W. (2007). *The Horse, The Wheel and Language: How Bronze-Age Riders from the Eurasian Steppes Shaped the Modern World.* Princeton, N.J.:Princeton University Press.

Anthony, D. W. (2009). *The Sintashta Genesis: The Roles of Climate Change, Warfare, and Long-Distance Trade. In* Hanks, B.; Linduff, K. *Social Complexity in Prehistoric Eurasia: Monuments, Metals, and Mobility.* Cambridge, U.K.: Cambridge University Press.

Apperson, C.S., Engber, B., Nicholson,W.L., Mead, D.G., & Engel, J. (2008). Tick-borne diseases in North Carolina: is *Rickettsia amblyommii* a possible cause of rickettsiosis reported as Rocky Mountain spotted fever? *Vector Borne Zoonotic Disease,* 8: 597–606.

Arvikar, S.L., Crowley, J.T., Sulka, K.B., & Steere, A.C. (2016). Autoimmune Arthritis, Rheumatoid Arthritis, Psoriatic Arthritis, or Peripheral Spondyloarthropathy, Following Lyme Disease. *Arthritis & Rheumatology.*

Attwell, L., Kovarovic, K., & Kendal, J.R. (2015). Fire in the Plio-Pleistocene: the functions of hominin fire use, and the mechanistic, developmental and evolutionary consequences. *Journal of Anthropological Sciences,* 93:1-20.

Auwaerter, P. MD, Bakken, J. MD, Dattwyler, R. MD, Dumler MD, Halperin, J.MD, McSweegan, E.PhD, Nadelman, R MD, O'Connell, S. MD, Shapiro, E.MD, Sood, S. MD, Steere, A. MD, Weinstein, A MD, Wormster, G.MD. (2011, September). Anti-science and ethical concerns associated with advocacy of Lyme disease. *The Lancet,* 9: 713–719.

Balashov, Y. S. (1994).Importance of continental drift in the distribution and evolution of Ixodid ticks. *Entomological Review,* 73: 42-49.

Barbour AG. & Fish, D (1993) The biological and social phenomenon of Lyme disease. *Science* 260: 1610–1616.

Barbour,A.G. & Garon, C.F.(1987).Linear plasmids of the bacterium Borrelia burgdorferi have covalently closed ends. *Science,* 237:409–11.

Barbour, AG.(1988). Plasmid analysis of Borrelia burgdorferi, the Lyme disease agent. *Journal Clinical Microbiology,* 26:475–8.

Barquet, N & Domingo, P. (1997). Smallpox: the triumph over the most terrible of the ministers of death." *Annals of Internal Medicine,* 127, 8.1: 635–42.

Bauman, N. (2014, February 3).Genes Linked to SLE, IL-18 Imported From Neanderthals. *Musculoskeletal Citations.*

Begley, S. (2017, October 5).Scientists introduce a new Neanderthal ancestor. You may be more related than you think. Neanderthal gene is associated with vitamin D (the rs6730714 variant of the PAX3 gene). *STAT.*

Bellomo, R. V. (1994, July 1). methods of determining early hominid behavioral activities associated with the controlled use of fire, Koobi Fora, Kenya. *Journal of Human Evolution,*27, 1–3:173-195.

Benedict, C.(1996). *Bubonic Plague in Nineteenth-century China.* Stanford, CA: Stanford University Press.

Bhandoo, S. (2012, June 28). Remnants of Ancient Kitchen found in China. *The New York Times.*

Blackmore, R.D.(1866). *A Tale of the New Forest,* Vol. 1. London: Chapman and Hall.

Bower, B. (2017, July 14). Copper in Ötzi the Iceman's ax came from surprisingly far away. Analysis hints that long-distance trade network connected present-day central and northern Italy. *ScienceNews.*

Bowman, A.S. & Sauer, J.R. (2004). Tick salivary glands: function, physiology and future. *Parasitology,*129, Suppl:S67-81.

Bowman,D., Balch, J., Artaxo, P., Bond, W.,Cochrane, M., D'Antonio, C., DeFries, R., Johnston, F., Keeley, J. (2011, December).The human dimension of fire regimes on Earth. Journal Biogeography, 38,12: 2223–2236.

Braitseva, OA, Melekestsev, IV, Sulerzhitskiy LD. (2004). Catastrophic eruptions of Avachinsky volcano (Kamchatka) in Holocene: chronology, dynamics, geological and geomorphological effect, environmental impact and long-term forecast. *Volcanol Seismology* 6: 3-8 [in Russian].

Bridges, P. S. (1991). Degenerative Joint Disease in Hunter-Gatherers and Agriculturalists from the Southeastern United States. *American Journal of Physical Anthropology* 85: 379-391.

Bridges, P.S. (1992). Prehistoric Arthritis in the Americas. *Annual Review of Anthropology* 21: 67- 91.

Brownstein, J.S., Holford,T., & Fish, D. (2005, March). Effect of Climate Change on Lyme Disease Risk in North America. *Ecohealth*, 2,1: 38–46.

Brustolin, S., Giugliani, R., Félix, T.M. (2010).Genetics of homocysteine metabolism and associated disorders. *Braz J Med Bir Res*. 43: 1–7.

Buhner, S.H. (2005). Healing Lyme. *Natural Healing and Prevention of Lyme Borreliosis and its Coinfections*. Raven Press.

Capasso, L. (1998, December). 5300 years ago, the Ice Man used natural laxatives and antibiotics. *Lancet* 352, 9143: 1864.

Carlyon,J.A.,Roberts,D.M.,Theisen,M., & Marconi, R.T.(1999). Molecular analyses of the B. turicatae bdr genes: a polymorphic, linear plasmid carried, paralogous gene family. *Emerging Infectious Diseases,*6, 2.

Carlyon, J.A., Roberts , D.M. & Marconi R.T. (2000) Evolutionary and molecular analyses of the Borrelia rep super gene family: delineation of six distinct sub-families and demonstration of the genus wide conservation of putative functional domains, structural properties and repeat motifs. *Microb Pathology*.

Carter, R. & Mendis, K.N.(2002, October). Evolutionary and Historical Aspects of the Burden of Malaria. *Clinical Microbiology Reviews,* 15,4:564-594.

Casjens, S. (1999, October). Evolution of the linear DNA replicons of the Borrelia spirochetes. *Curr Opin Microbiol,* 2,5:529-34.

Cavalli-Sforza, L.L. & Minch, E.(1997, July). Paleolithic and Neolithic lineages in the European mitochondrial gene pool. *Am J Hum Genetics.*

Chary-Valckenaere, I., Guillemin, F., Pourel,J., Schiele, F., Heller, R.& Jaulhac, B. (1997). Seropositivity to Borrelia Burgdorferi antigens in early rheumatoid arthritis: A Case Control Study. *British Journal of Rheumatology*,36:945-949.

Chaudhry A. R., Chaudhry M. R., Papadimitriou J. C., Drachenberg C. B. (2015).Bartonella henselae infection-associated vasculitis and crescentic glomerulonephritis leading to renal allograft loss. *Transplant Infectious Disease*,17, 3:411–417.

Chen, L.F. & Sexton, D.J. (2008).What's new in Rocky Mountain spotted fever? *Dis Clin North Am.* Sep,22,3:415-32.

Chicki, L.The Neolithic Transition and the Genetics of Populations in Europe. Princeton, N.J.: Princeton University Press.

Chicki, L., Nichols, R.A., Barbujani, G. & Beaumont, M.A. (2002). Y genetic data support the Neolithic demic diffusion model. *Proc. Natl. Acad. Sci.* 99,17: 11008-11013.

Chiuri R. M., Matronola M. F., Di Giulio C., Comegna L., Chiarelli F., Blasetti A.(2013). Bartonella henselae infection associated with autoimmune thyroiditis in a child. *Hormone Research in Paediatrics,* 79, 3:185–188.

Choi, C. (2017, March 8). Ailing Neanderthals Used Penicillin and 'Aspirin'. *Discovery Magazine.*

Chomel, B.B. & Boulouis, H.J. (2005). Zoonotic diseases caused by bacteria of the genus *Bartonella*: new reservoirs? new vectors?" *Bulletin Academy National Medicine* (in French).189, 3: 465–77; discussion 477–80.

Chouikha, I. & Hinnebusch, B. J. (2014, December). Silencing urease: A key evolutionary step that facilitated the adaptation of *Yersinia pestis* to the flea-borne transmission route. *PNAS* 111, 52:18709–18714.

Chua, L., Rahaman, N., Adnan, N. & Eddie Tan, T. (2013). Antioxidant Activity of Three Honey Samples in relation with Their Biochemical Components. *J Anal Methods Chemistry*.
Cilek, J. & Olson, M .(2000). Seasonal distribution and abundance of ticks (Acari: Ixodidae) in northwestern Florida. *J Med Entomol* 37: 439–444.

Clark, L. & Rawcliffe, C., Eds. (2013). *Society in the Age of Plague*. London, U.K.:Boydell Press.

Columbia University Medical Center (2017). Lyme and Tick-borne Diseases Research Center.

Conner, D.W.(2017, November 15). Lyme Disease Patients File Federal Antitrust Suit Against Infectious Disease Specialists & Health Insurers. *The Huffington Post*.

Cosentino, S., Tubeerso, C., Pisano, B., Satta, M., Mascia, V., Arzedi, E., Palmas,F. (1999).In- Vitro Antimicrobial Activity and Chemical Composition of Sardinian Thymus Essential Oils. *Lett Appl Microbiol,* 29:130–135.

Croft, L. R. (1989). *Curiosities of Beekeeping*. Campbell, CA?.: Elmwood.

Cronin, W. (2003). *Changes in the Land*. New York: Hill & Wang.

Cully, J. (1999). Lone star tick abundance, fire, and bison grazing in tallgrass prairie. *J Range Manag*e 52: 139–144.

Daley, B. (2013, December 3). Physician embodies puzzle of Lyme diseaseTodd Murray has suffered from Lyme-related symptoms for four decades. His mother, Polly Murray, sounded the original alarm about Lyme disease back in the '70s. *The Boston Globe.*

Danneman, M., Andrés, A., Kelso, J. (2016, January 7). Introgression of Neandertal- and Denisovan-like Haplotypes Contributes to Adaptive Variation in Human Toll-like Receptors. *AJHG,*98,1: 22–33.

Dannemann, M. & Kelso, J. (2017, October 5). Contribution of Neanderthals to Phenotypic Variation in Modern Humans. *American Journal of Human Genetics,*101,4:578–589.

Davidson, W.R., Siefkan, D.A., Creekmore, L.H. (1994). Influence of annual and biennial prescribed burning during March on the abundance of *Amblyomma americanum* (Acari: Ixodidae) in central Georgia. *J Med Entomol,* 31: 72–81.

Deans, S.G. & Ritchie, G.A. (1987). Antimicrobial properties of plant essential oils. *Int J Food Microbiology,* 5:165–180.

Delcourt P.A., Delcourt H.R. (1992). Ecotone Dynamics in Space and Time. In: Hansen A.J., Castri F. (Eds). Landscape Boundaries. *Ecological Studies,* 92. New York, N.Y.: Springer.

Denevan, W.M. (1992, September).The Pristine Myth: The Landscape of the Americas in 1492. *Annals of the Association of American Geographers.*

Dennell, R. & Petraglia, M. D. (2012). The dispersal of Homo sapiens across southern Asia: how early, how often, how complex?. *Quaternary Science Reviews,* 47: 15–22.

Dennell, R. (2015, October 14). Palaeoanthropology: Homo sapiens in China 80,000 years ago. *Nature,* 526: 647–648.

Derbyshire, D. (2002, May 20). Discovery of grave may solve mystery death of Henry VIII's brother at 15. *BST.*

Deschamps,M., Laval,G., Fagny,M., Itan,Y., Abel, L., Casanova,J-L., Patin,E., Quintana-Murci,L. (2016, January 7). Genomic Signatures of Selective Pressures and Introgression from Archaic Hominins at Human Innate Immunity Genes.*AJHG,* 98,1:5–21.

Deter-Wolf, A., Robitaile, B., Krutak & L.,Galliot, S. (2015). The World's Oldest Tattoos. *Journal of Archaeological Science.*
Dever, L.L., Jorgensen, J.H. & Barbour, A.G.(1993). In vitro activity of vancomycin against the spirochete Borrelia burgdorferi. *Antimicrobal Agents Chemotherapy,* 37,5:1115-1121.

Dharmananda, S.(June 1999) *Lyme disease: Treatment with Chinese Herbs.* Portland, Oregon: Institute for Traditional Medicine.

Diamond, J. (1997). *Guns, Germs, and Steel: The Fates of Human Societies.* New York: W.W. Norton.

Dickson, K. (2015). Dearborn Happened to Hide Neurologic Disease from LYMErix. *www.actionlyme.com.*

Didier Raoult, D.& Drancourt, M, Eds. (2008). *Paleomicrobiology of Humans.* American Society of Paleomicrobiology.

Dilworth, C. (2010).*Too Smart for Our Own Good: The Ecological Predicament of Humankind.* Cambridge, UK: Cambridge University Press.

Dodson ,J., & Dong ,G.. (2016). What do we know about domestication in eastern Asia? *Quaternary International,* 426:2-9.

Dolan, M., Lacomb,E.,Piesman, J. (2000).Vector competence of Ixodes angustus (Acari: Ixodidae) for Borrelia burgdorferi ss. *Experimental and Applied Acarology*, 24,1:77-84.

Donalson, M. D. (1999). *The Domestic Cat in Roman Civilization*. Lewiston, New York: The Edwin Mellen Press.

Doppler, T., Gerling, C., Heye, V. & Schibler,J. (2015, October) Landscape opening and herding strategies: Carbon isotope analyses of herbivore bone collagen from the Neolithic and Bronze Age lakeshore site of Zurich-Mozartstrasse, Switzerland. *Quaternary International*.

Drancourt, M., Tran-Hung, L., Courtin, J., Lumley, H.& Raoult, D. (2005). *Bartonella quintana* in a 4000- year-old human tooth. *Journal Infect. Dis,*191,4: 607–11.

Drew, M., Samuel, W., Lukiwski, G. & Willman, J. (1985). An evaluation of burning for control of winter ticks, *Dermacentor albipictus*, in central Alberta. *J Wildl Dis,* 21: 313–315.

Driscoll, C., Marilyn Menotti-Raymond, M., Roca, A., Hupe, K., Johnson, W., , Geffen, E. , Harley, E., Delibes, M., Pontier, D. Kitchener, A., Yamaguchi, N., O'Brien, S., Macdonald, D.(2007, July 27).The Near Eastern Origin of Cat Domestication. *Science* 317,3837:519-23.

Driscoll, C., Clutton-Brock, J., Kitchener, A. & O'Brien, S. (2009, June). The Taming of the Cat. *Scientific American,* 300, 68 – 75.

Drymon, M.M. (2008). *Disguised as the Devil: How Lyme disease Created Witches and Changed History.* Brooklyn, N.Y. :Wythe Avenue Press.

Dueppen, S. (2011, March). Early evidence for chickens at Iron Age Kirikongo (c. AD 100– 1450), Burkina Faso. *Antiquity*,85, 327:142-157.

Dworkin, M.S., Schwan, T.G., Anderson, D.E., Jr, Borchardt, S.M. (2008). Tick-borne relapsing fever. *Infect Dis Clin North Am.* 22, 3:449-68.

Eiger-Moscovich M., Amer R., Oray M., Tabbara K. F., Tugal-Tutkun I., Kramer M. (2016). Retinal artery occlusion due to Bartonella henselae infection: a case series. *Acta Ophthalmologica*, 94, 5:e367–e370.

Ellis, G. (1848). *Specimens of Early English Metrical Romances.* London, U.K.

Embury-Dennis,T. (2017, October 19). Prehistoric Teeth Fossils dating back 9.7 million years could re-write human history. *The Independent.*

Elton, S. (2008, April). The environmental context of human evolutionary history in Eurasia and Africa. *Journal Anatomy* 212, 4: 377–393.

Engels, D.W. (1999). *Classical Cats: The Rise and Fall of the Sacred Cat.* Psychology Press.
Erbstösser, M.(1978). *The Crusades.* Brunel House, UK: David and Charles.

Eustace, C. (2006, April 24).Cytokines. *BioBasics.*

Egyed, L. (2017, June). Difference in susceptibility of small rodent host species to infestation by Ixodes ricinus larvae. *Experimental and Applied Acarology,* 72, 2: 183–189.

Faber, A., Hornig, H., Jungklaus, B., Niemitz, C. (2003).Age structure and selected pathological aspects of a series of skeletons of late medieval Bernau (Brandenburg, Germany). *Anthropol Anz,.* 61, 1: 89-202.

Eskow, E., Rao, R.V.,Mordechai,E.(2001).Concurrent Infection of the Central Nervous System by Borrelia burgdorferi and Bartonella henselae: Evidence for a Novel Tick-borne Disease Complex. *Arch Neurol,* 58, 9:1357-1363.

Fagan, B. (2006). *Fish on Friday: Feasting, Fasting, and Discovery of the New World.* New York: Basic Books.

Falkow, S.,Rosenberg,E., Schleifer, K-H., Stackebrandt, E. (2006, November 14).The Prokaryotes: Vol. 7: Proteobacteria: Delta and Epsilon Subclasses. Deeply Rooting Bacteria. *Springer Science & Business Media.*

Fallon, B.,Nields, J. M.D., Burrascano, J., Leigner, K., Donato DelBene, D., Liebowitz, M.(1992).The Neuropsychiatric Manifestations of Lyme Borreliosis. *Psychiatric Quarterly,*63, 1.

Faure, E & Kitchener, A.(2009). An Archaeological and Historical Review of the Relationships between Felids and People. *Anthrozoos,* 22: 221-238.

Feng, J., Zhang, S.,Shi,W.,Zubcevik, N. Miklossy, J & Zhang, Y. (2017, October 11). Selective Essential Oils from Spice or Culinary Herbs Have High Activity against Stationary Phase and Biofilm Borrelia burgdorferi. *Frontiers in Medicine.*

Ferdows, M.S. & Barbour, A.G.(1989). Megabase-sized linear DNA in the bacterium Borrelia burgdorferi, the Lyme disease agent. *PNAS,* 86:5969–73.

Fernández, P. J., González, V.B., Blasco, R, Cuartero, F., Fluck, H, Sañudo, P, & Verdasco, C. (2012). The earliest evidence of hearths in Southern Europe: The case of Bolomor Cave (Valencia, Spain). *Quaternary International.*

Fernandes, P.M. & Botehlo, H.S. (2003). A review of prescribed burning effectiveness in fire hazard reduction. *Int J Wildland Fire* 12: 117–128.

Ferretti, A., Parisi ,P., Villa, M.P. (2013).The role of hyperhomocysteinemia in neurological features associated with celiac disease. *Med Hypotheses*, 81: 524–31.

Fix, A., Peña, C., Strickland, G.T. (2000, October). Racial Differences in Reported Lyme Disease Incidence. *American Journal of Epidemiology*, 152, 8:756–759.

Foster, D.R. & O'Keefe, J.F. (2000). *New England Forests Through Time: Insights from the Harvard Forest Dioramas.* Cambridge, Mass.: Harvard University Press.

Fowler, B. (2001). *Iceman: Uncovering the Life and Times of a Prehistoric Man found in an Alpine Glacier*, Chicago, Ill.: University of Chicago Press.

Frater, H.E. (2011). Impact of prescribed burning for oak regeneration on forest vegetation, white-footed mouse populations, and Lyme disease. *M.S. Thesis.* Iowa State University, Iowa.

Fukunaga, M., Okada, K., Naka, M., Konishi, T., Sato, Y. (1996, October). Phylogenetic Analysis of Borrelia Species Based on Flagellin Gene Sequences and Its Application for MolecularTyping of Lyme Disease Borreliae. *Journal of Systematic Bacteriology*, 46, 4: 898-905.

Furuse, Y., Suzuki, A., Oshitani, H. (2010, March 4).Origin of measles virus: divergence from rinderpest virus between the 11th and 12th centuries. *Virology Journal.*

Gannon, M.(2017, October 23). Europe's Oldest Battlefield Yields Clues to Fighter's Identities. *ScienceLive.*

Gavashelishvili, A. & Tarkhnishvili, D. (2016). Biomes and human distribution during the last ice age. *Global Ecology and Biogeography,* 25: 563–74.

Geoffrey, E. (2016, April 24).Fighting ticks with fire: A health benefit from forest management. http://www.georgiahealthnews.com.

Georgievska, M. (2017, February 6). In the Middle Ages, devil-fearing Christians killed cats, which carried the unintended consequence of increasing the rat population and the spread of the Black Death. *Vintage News.*

Gibbons, A. (2014, September 4). Three-part ancestry for Europeans. *Science.* American Association for the Advancement of Science.

Gibbons, A. (2017, February 21). Thousands of horsemen may have swept into Bronze Age Europe, transforming the local population. *Science.* American Association for the Advancement of Science.

Gibson, M.,Young, C., Omran, J.,Edwards, K.,Palma, L.Russell, L. & Rawlings, J. (1993). *Borrelia burgdorferi* infection of cats. *Journal American Vet Med Association*, 202,1786.

Gleim, E.R., Conner, L.M., Berghaus, R., Levin, M., Zemtsova, G.,Yabsley, M.(2014, November 6).The Phenology of Ticks and the Effects of Long-Term Prescribed Burning on Tick Population Dynamics in Southwestern Georgia and Northwestern Florida. *PLOS ONE* 9,11.

Goddard, J., Embers,M., Hojgaard,A., & Piesman, J.(2015, January).Comparison of Tick Feeding Success and Vector Competence for Borrelia burgdorferi Among Immature Ixodes scapularis (Ixodida: Ixodidae) of Both Southern and Northern Clades. *J Med Entomol*, 52,1: 81–85.

Goldberg, A., Gunther, T., Rosenberg, N., Jakobsson, M. (2017, February 21). Ancient X chromosomes reveal contrasting sex bias in Neolithic and Bronze Age Eurasian migrations. *PNAS* 114,10: 2657–2662.

Goodin, D.G., Koch, D.E., Owen, R.D., Chu, Y., Hutchinson, J. (2006). Land cover associated with hantavirus presence in Paraguay. *Global Ecol Biogeography,* 15: 519–527.

Gowlett, J.,& Wrangham, R.W. (2013).Earliest fire in Africa: towards the convergence of archaeological evidence and the cooking hypothesis. *Azania: Archaeological Research in Africa* 48,1:5-30.

Gowlett, J. (2016, June 5). The Discovery of fire by humans: a long and convoluted process. *Transaction of the Royal Society B:* 371.

Green, M. H.; Symes, C., Colet, A., Suntané i Santiveri, J., Xavier; R., Saula, O., Subirà de Galdàcano, M., Jáuregui, C., DeWie, S., Borsch, S., Carmichael, A., Varlık, N., Crespo, F., Lawrenz, M., Ziegler, M., Hymes, R., Walker-Meikle, K., & Müller, W. P. (2014). *Pandemic Disease in the Medieval World: Rethinking the Black Death.* TMG.

Greiner, E., Humphrey, P.,Belden,R.,Frankenberger, W, Austin, D., & Gibbs, E.P. (1984). *Ixodid* ticks on feral swine in Florida. *Journal of Wildlife Diseases.*

Guerra, M., Walker, E., Jones,C., Paskewitz, S., Roberto Cortinas, M., Stancil, A., Beck, L., Bobo, M., & Kitron, U. (2002, March). Predicting the Risk of Lyme Disease: Habitat Suitability for Ixodes scapularis in the North Central United States. *Emerging Infectious Diseases,* 8, 3.

Gustafson, E. (2002). Evaluation of spatial Modesto predict vulnerability of forest birds to proof parasitism. *Ecological Applications,* 12, 2:412-426.

Hadid, Y. (2017). *Believe Me: My Battle with the Invisible Disability of Lyme Disease.* New York: St. Martins Press.

Haines, T.K., Busby R.L., Cleaves D.L. (2001). Prescribed burning in the South: Trends, purposes, and barriers. *Southern J. Appl. Forestry* 25: 149–153.

Holloway, A. (2013, December 30).Chinese May Have Loved Cats before Ancient Egyptians. *Ancient Origins.*

Harman, M.W., Hamby, A.E., Boltyanskiy, R., Belperron, A.A., Bockenstedt, L.K., Kress, H., Dufresne, E.R., Wolgemuth, C.W. (2017).Vancomycin Reduces Cell Wall Stiffness and Slows Swim Speed of the Lyme Disease Bacterium. *Biophysical Journal*, 112,4: 746-754.

Haydak, M. (1942). *Honey,and the vitamin content of thirty-one individual samples of honey from v a r i o u s   r e g i o n s   o f territorialUnited States as well as seven samples of foreign honey.*Washington, D.C.: United States Department of Agriculture.

Hein, S., Agnetha, H., Fedor, G., Willem, T., Frans, J., van Vliet, AJH, van Ballegooijen, M., van der Giessen, J., Katsuhisa T. (2012). Circumstantial evidence for an increase in the total number and activity of borrelia-infected *Ixodes ricinus* in the Netherlands. *Parasites & Vectors*, 5: 294.

Heiss, A.G. & Oeggl, K. (2008, February 19). The plant macro-remains from the Iceman site (Tisenjoch, Italian-Austrian border, eastern Alps): new results on the glacier mummy's environment. *Veget Hist Archaeobot*,18: 23–35.

Hesketh, T., Ye, X.J., Zhu, W.X. (2008, June 20). Syphilis in China: the great comeback. *Health Threats,* 1: e6.

Hinnebusch, J. & Barbour, A.G.(1991). Linear plasmids of Borrelia burgdorferi have a telomeric structure and sequence similar to those of a eukaryotic virus. *Journal Bacteriology,* 173:7233–39.

Hillier, L., Miller, W.,Birney, E.,Warren,W., Hardison,R., Ponting,C.P., Bork,P., Burt,D., Groenen, M.,Delany, M., Dodgson, J. (2004, December 9).Sequence and comparative analysis of the chicken genome provide unique perspectives on vertebrate evolution. *Nature* 432: 695-716.

Hoen, A., Margos, G., Bent, S., Diuk-Wasser, M., Barbour, A., Kurtenbach, K., & Fish, D. (2009). Phylogeography of Borrelia burgdorferi in the easternUnited States reflects multiple independent Lymedisease emergence events. *PNAS*.

Hong, J., Li ,Y., Hua, X., Bai ,Y., Wang, C., Zhu, C., Du, Y., Yang, Z., Yuan, C.(2017, January). Lymphatic Circulation Disseminates Bartonella Infection Into Bloodstream. *J Infect Dis.215, 2:303-311.*

Houzel, S.H. (2016).*The Human Advantage: A New Understanding of How Our Brain Became Remarkable*. MIT Press.

Holden, T.G. (2002). The Food Remains from the Colon of the Tyrolean Ice Man: 35-40, in Dobney, K.& O'Connor,T.,Ed. *Bones and the Man: Studies in Honour of Don Brothwell.* Oxford: Oxbow Books.

Horowitz, R.(2013). *Why can't I get better. Solving the Mystery of Lyme and Chronic disease.* St. Martins Press. New York:New York.

Hou, P-W., Fu, P-K., Hsu, H-C., Hsieh, C-L. (2015, October).Traditional Chinese medicine in patients with osteoarthritis of the knee. *J Tradit Complement Med*icine, 5,4: 182–196.

Houldcroft, C. & Underdown, S. (2016).Neanderthal Genomics suggest a Pleistocene Time Frame for the First Epidemiological Transition. *American Journal of Physical Anthropology*, 160: 379-388.

Hsieh,Y-F., Liu,H-W.,Hsu, T-C.,Wei, J., Shih,C-M.,Krause, P. & Tsay, G. (2007, November). Serum Reactivity against Borrelia burgdorferi OspA in Patients with Rheumatoid Arthritis. *Clin Vaccine Immunology,* 14,11: 1437–1441.

Hu, Y., Hu, S., Huc, W., Wud, X., Marshalle,F., Chena,X.,Houa,L., & Wanga, C. (2013, November 13). Earliest evidence for commensal processes of cat domestication. *PNAS* 111, 1:116–120.

Hu, Y., Shangc, H., Tong, H., Nehlich, O., Liu, W., Zhao, C., Yuf, J., Wang, C., Trinkaus, E., Richards, M.(2009) Stable isotope dietary analysis of the Tianyuan 1 early modern human. *PNAS,* 106, 27: 10971–10974.

Hummel, S.,Schmidt, D. & Hutton W. (1813).*The Battle of Bosworth Field between Richard the Third and Henry Earl of Richmond August 22,1485.* Nichols, Son, and Bentley; London, UK.

Ibáñez, V. B. (1916). *The Four Horsemen of the Apocalypse.* film.

Innes, J.B. & Blackford, J.J. (2003, February). The Ecology of Late Mesolithic Woodland Disturbances: Model Testing with Fungal Spore Assemblage Data. *Journal of Archaeological Science* 30, 2: 185-194

Inoue, K., Hukuda, S., Fardellon, P., Yang, Z., Nakai, M., Katayama, K., Ushiyama, T., Saruhashi, Y., Huang, J., Mayeda, A. (2001, January 1)Prevalence of large−joint osteoarthritis in Asian and Caucasian skeletal populations. *Rheumatology,* 40, 1:70–73.

Jennett, A., Smith, F.& Wall, R. (2013). Tick infestation risk for dogs in a peri-urban park. *Parasites & Vectors,* 6:358.

Johanson, D. C. & Wong, K. (2010). *Lucy's Legacy: The Quest for Human Origins.* New York: Crown Publishing Group.

Johnson, L., Wilcox, S., Mankoff, J., & Stricker, R. (2014, March 27). Severity of chronic Lyme disease compared to other chronic conditions: a quality of life survey. *Peer J.*

Jones, C. & Kitron, U.D.(2000). Populations of Ixodes Scapularis are modulated by drought at a Lyme disease focus in Illinois. *Journal Med Entomology,* 37: 408-415.

Kaf-Ngoane, S. (2006,August 23). Lyme disease: the forgotten scourge of West Africa. www.irinnews.org

Kaplan, J. O., Krumhardt, K.M. & Zimmermann, N.(2009). The prehistoric and preindustrial deforestation of Europe.*Quaternary Science Reviews,* 28, 3016–3034.

Kaplan, J.O., Pfeiffer, M., Kolen,J.& Davis, B.(2016, November 30).Large Scale Anthropogenic Reduction of Forest Cover in Last Glacial Maximum Europe. *PLOS ONE.*

Karkanas P., Shahack-Gross, R., Ayalon, A., Bar-Matthews, M., Barkai, R., Frumkin, A., Gopher. A., & Stiner, M.C. (2007).Evidence for habitual use of fire at the end of the Lower Paleolithic: Site-formation processes at Qesem Cave, Israel. *Journal of Human Evolution*,53,2:197-212.

Kean, W., Tocchio, S., Kean, M., & Rainsford, K.D.(2013, February).The musculoskeletal abnormalities of the Similaun Iceman ("ÖTZI"): clues to chronic pain and possible treatments. *Inflammopharmacology* 21,1:11–20

Keller, A. Graefen, A., Ball, M., Matzas, M., Boisguerin, V., Maixner, F., Leidinger, P., Backes, C., Khairat, R., Forster, M., Stade, B., Franke, A., Mayer, J., Spangler, J., McLaughlin, S., Shah, M., Lee, C., Harkins, T., Sartori, A., Moreno-Estrada, A., Henn, B., Sikora, M., Semino, O., Chiaroni, J., Rootsi, S., Myres, N., Cabrera, V., Underhill, P., Bustamante, C., Vigl, E., Samadelli, M., Cipollini, G., Haas, J., Katus, H., O'Connor, B., Carlson, M., Meder, B., Blin, N., Meese, E., Pusch, C., & Zink, A. (2012, February 28). New insights into the Tyrolean Iceman's origin and phenotype as inferred by whole-genome sequencing. *Nature Communications,* 3: 698.

Kilpatrick, A.M., Dobson, A.D.M., Levi, T., Salkeld, D., Swei, A., Ginsberg, H., Kjemtrup,, A.,Padgett, K., Jensen, P., Fish,D.,Ogden, N.,and Diuk-Wasser, M. (2017, April 24). Lyme disease ecology in a changing world: consensus, uncertainty and critical gaps for improving control. *Transactions of The Royal Society B.*

Klitza, W., Brautbar, C., Schito, A.,Barcellos. L.,Roksenberg, J. (2001, May 5).Evolution of the CCR5 δ32 mutation based on haplotype variation in Jewish and Northern European population samples. *Human Immunology,* 62, 5: 530-538.

Klompen, J. S.& Grimaldi, D. (2001). First Mesozoic record of a Parasitifom mite: a larval Argasid tick in Cretaceousamber (Acari: Ixodida, Argasida). *Annals of Entomological Society of America,* 94:10-15.

Kramar C., Lagier, R., Baud, C.A.(1990, Nov.-Dec.). Rheumatic diseases in Neolithic and Medieval populations of western Switzerland. *Z Rheumatol,*49,6:338-45.

Krause, P.J., Feder, H.M., Jr. (1994) Lyme disease and babesiosis. *Adv Pediatr Infect* Dis, 9: 183-209.

Kristiansen, K., Allentoft, Frei, Iversen, Johannsen, Kroonen, Pospiezny, Price, Rasmussen, Sjögren, Sikora & Willerslev, E. (2017, April 4). Re-theorising mobility and the formation of culture and language among the Corded Ware Culture in Europe. *Antiquity.*

Kröber, T. & Guerin, P.M. (1999, July). Ixodid ticks avoid contact with liquid water. *Journal of Experimental Biology,* 202:1877-1883.

Kuhn, S., Stiner, M., Gulec, E., Ozer, I., Yilmaz,H.,Baykara,I.,Acikkol, A.,Goldberg,P., Molina,K.,Uney, E. (2009). The Early Upper Paleolithic Occupation at Ucaqlzli Cave. *Journal of Human Evolution*, 56:87-113.

Kuper, R. & Kröpelin, S.(2006, August 11).Climate-Controlled Holocene Occupation in the Sahara: Motor of Africa's Evolution. *Science*, 313, 5788: 803-807.

La, V.D., Clavel, B., Lepetz, S., Aboudharam, G., Raoult, D.& Drancourt,M. (2004).Molecular detection of Bartonella henselae DNA in the dental pulp of 800-year-old French cats. *Clin Infect Dis*ease, 39:1391-1394.

Laayouni, H., Oosting, M., Luisia, P., Ioanab,M.,Alonsoe, S., Ricaño-Poncef, I.,Trynkaf,G., Zhernakovaf, A., Plantinga, T., Shih-Chin Cheng, S-C.,van der Meer,J., Poppg, R., Soodh,A., Thelmai, B., Wijmengaf,C., Joostenb,L., Bertranpetita, J., & Neteab,M. (2014, February 18). Convergent evolution in European and Roma populations reveals pressure exerted by plague on Toll-like receptors. *PNAS,* 111, 7: 2668-2673.

Lagier, R. (2006, March). Bone eburnation in rheumatic diseases: a guiding trace in today's radiological diagnosis and in paleopathology. *Clin Rheumatol*, 25,2:127-31.

Lamb,H., Gasse,F., Benkaddour,A., El Hamouti,N., Van Der Kaars, S., Perkins, W.,Pearce, & Roberts, C.(1995).Relation between century-scale Holocene arid intervals in tropical and temperate zones. *Nature,* 373: 134 .

Landford, C. (2017, November 14). Insurers Accused of Conspiring to Deny Lyme Disease Coverage. *www.courthousenews.com.*

Lane, R.S. & Quistad, G.B. (Feb., 1998, February) Borreliacidal Factor in the Blood of the Western Fence Lizard (Sceloporus occidentalis).*The Journal of Parasitology,* 84, 1:29-34.

Lathem, W.W., Price, P.,Miller, V.,Goldman, W. (2007, January 26). A Plasminogen-Activating Protease Specifically Controls the Development of Primary Pneumonic Plague. *Science,* 315, 5811: 509-513

Lawlor, A. & Adler, J. (2012, June). How the Chicken Conquered the World:The epic begins 10,000 years ago in an Asian jungle and ends today in kitchens all over the world. *Smithsonian Magazine.*

LeBlanc, J.G., Milani,C., de Giori, G.S., Sesma, F., van Sinderen, D., Ventura, M. (2012, August). Bacteria as vitamin suppliers to their host: a gut microbiota perspective. *Current Opinion in Biotechnology,* 24, 2.

Ledford, H. (2008, July 16). African mutation may increase HIV infectionGenetic quirk fends off malaria, but may render Africans more vulnerable to HIV. *Nature.*

Lehane,M.J.(1991). *Biology of Blood-Sucking Insects.* Harper Collins: London, UK.

Lehman, H. E. (2011). *Lives of England's Reigning and Consort Queens.* AuthorHouse Publishing.

Lewis, B. A. (1991). Analysis of Pathologies Present in the 16ST1 Tchefuncte Indian Skeletal Collection. *M.A. Thesis*, Louisiana State University.

Lewis, B.A.(1994). Treponematosis and Lyme Borreliosis Connections: Explanations for Tchefuncte Disease Syndromes? *American Journal of Physical Anthropology,* 93:455-475.

Lewis, B.A.(1998). Prehistoric Juvenile Rheumatoid Arthritis in a Precontact Louisiana Native Population Reconsidered. *American Journal of Physical Anthropology,* 106: 229-248.

Li, H., Bai, J.Y., Wang, L.Y., Zeng, L., Shi,Y.S., Qiu, Z.L., Ye, H.H,. Zhang, X.F., Lu, Q.B., Kosoy, M., Liu, W., & Cao, W.C. (2013). Genetic diversity of Bartonella quintana in macaques suggests zoonotic origin of trench fever. *Molecular Ecology*, 22, 8: 2118-27.

License, A. (2016). *Catherine of Aragon: An Intimate Life of Henry VIII's True Wife.* Amberley Publishing Limited.
Little, L., Ed. (2007). *Plague and the End of Antiquity: The Pandemic of 541-750.* Cambridge, U.K.: Cambridge University Press.

Lutz, H.,Engel, T., Lischewsky, B., Von Berg, A.(2017, October). A new great ape with startling resemblances to African members of the hominin tribe, excavated from the Mid-Vallesian Dinotheriensande of Eppelsheim. *First report* (Hominoidea, Miocene, MN 9, Proto-Rhine River, Germany) 9.5 million years ago.

Ma, K-W.(2000). Acupuncture: Its Place in the History of Chinese Medicine. *British Medical Journal*, 18,2: 88-97.

Mallory, J. P., Mair, V. H. (2000). *The Tarim Mummies: Ancient China and the Mystery of the Earliest Peoples from the West.* London: Thames & Hudson.

Marquer L., Otto, T., Nespoulet, R., & Chiotti, L. (2010, November). A new approach to study the fuel used in hearths by hunter-gatherers at the Upper Palaeolithic site of Abri Pataud (Dordogne, France). *Journal of Archaeological Science*, 37,11:2735-2746.

Maeda, K., Markowitz, N., Hawley, R.C., Ristic,M., Cox, D. (1987). Human infection with *Ehrlichia canis*, a leukocytic rickettsia. *N Engl J Med*, 316: 853–856.

Maggi, R., Mozayeni, R., Pultorak,E., Hegarty, B., Bradley, J., Correa, M., & Breitschwert, E. (2012, May). Bartonella spp. Bacteremia and Rheumatic Symptoms in Patients from Lyme Disease–endemic Region. *Emerging Infectious Diseases*,18, 5.

Magnarelli LA, Anderson JF, Kaufmann AF, Lieberman LL, Whitney GD.(1985). Borreliosis in dogs from southern Connecticut. *J Am Vet Med Assoc*, 186: 955–959.

Maguina, C., Garcia, P.J., Gotuzzo, E., Cordero, L., Spach, D. (2001, September 15) Bartonelliosis (Carrión's Disease) in the Modern Era. *Clinical Infectious Diseases*, 33, 6:772–779.
Mandal, M. & Mandal,S. (2011, April). Honey: its medicinal property and antibacterial activity. *Asian Pac Journal Tropical Biomedicine,*1, 2:154-160.

Manella, M. (2016, April 15). Migrating humans may have killed off Neanderthals by accident. *CNN*.

Mans, B., de Klerk, D., Pienaar, R., & Latif, A. (2014, September 11). Nuttalliella namaqua: A Living Fossil and Closest Relative to the Ancestral Tick Lineage: Implications for the Evolution of Blood-Feeding in Ticks. *Experimental and Applied Acarology*, 62, 2: 233–240.

Marcus, S. (2015, June 29). Avril Lavigne Breaks Down During Interview About Lyme Disease. *The Huffington Post.*

Markowitz, L.E., Steere, A.C., Benach, J.L., Slade, J.D.& Broome, C.V. (1986, June 27). Lyme disease during pregnancy. *JAMA*,255, 24:3394-6.

Mather, T., Duffy, D. & Campbell, S. (1993). An unexpected result from burning vegetation to reduce Lyme disease transmission risks. *J Med Entomology,* 30: 642–645.

Mathews, J. (2011). *The Great Men of Christendom: The Failure of the Third Crusade.* M.A. Thesis, Western Kentucky University.

Matthews, L. (2014, January 7). Lyme Disease… in Chickens? Not Quite. www.lymediseaseguide.net

Matuschka, F.R., Ohlenbusch, A., Eiffert, H., Richter, D., Spielman, A. (1996, August). Characteristics of Lyme disease spirochetes in archived European ticks. *J Infect Dis.*174, 2:424-6.

McCormack, W.J., Parker, A.E.& O'Neill, L.A.(2009, October 14). Toll-like receptors and NOD-like receptors in rheumatic diseases. *Arthritis Res Ther*, 11, 5:243.

McCoy, J. (2003, August 5). Amy Tan, Ticked Off About Lyme. *The Washington Post.*

McInnes, I & Schett, G. (2007, June).Cytokines in the pathogenesis of rheumatoid arthritis. *Nature Immunology.*

Meng, X.H., Liu, Z.J., Huang, F.S. (2004). Ticks in China such as Lyme disease media research situation. *Health Helminthic Machinery,* 3: 137-140.

Michels, H. T., Wilks, S. A.& Keevil, C. W. (2003). The Antimicrobial Effects of Copper Alloy Surfaces on the Bacterium

E. coli. Proceedings of Copper 2003 - Cobre 2003, *The 5th International Conference, Santiago, Chile, Plenary Lectures, Economics and Applications of Copper*, Montreal, Quebec, Canada: The Canadian Institute of Mining, Metallurgy and Petroleum,1: 439–450.

Mirouse G., Journe A., Casabianca L., Moreau P. E., Pannier S., Glorion C.(2015). Bartonella henselae osteoarthritis of the upper cervical spine in a 14-year-old boy. *Orthopaedics & Traumatology: Surgery & Research,*101,4:519–522.

Mitchell, P. (2007). *Medicine in the Crusades: Warfare, Wounds and the Medieval Surgeon.* Cambridge, U.K.:Cambridge University Press.

MSNBC. (2009, July 17). *Otzi iceman's tattoos came from fireplace.*

Müller,W., Fricke,H.,Halliday, A.N., McCulloch, M.T., Wartho, J.A. (2003, October 31). Origin and Migration of the Alpine Iceman. *Science,*302,5646:862-6.

Mummert, A., Esche, E., Robinson,J. & Armelagos, G.J.(2011, July). Stature and robusticity during the agricultural transition: Evidence from the bioarchaeological record. *Economics and Human Biology.*

Murray, P. (1996). *The Widening Circle.* New York: St. Martin's Press.

Myolonis, I. (2011). Borreliosis During Pregnancy: A Risk for the Unborn Child? *Vector -Borne and Zoonotic Diseases,*11, 7: 891-898.

Narasimha, S., Schuijt,T., Abraham, N., Rajeevan, N., Coumou, J.,Graham, M.,Robson, A.Wu,M-J., Daffre, S., Hovius, J. & Fikrig, E.(2017).Modulation of the tick gut milieu by a secreted tick protein favors *Borrelia burgdorferi* colonization. *Nature.*

Ni, M. (1995). *The Yellow Emperor's Classic of Medicine: A New Translation of the Neijing Suwen.* Shambhala Press.

Ni, Q.L., Yin, H. & Luo, J.X. (2009). Progress on Lyme disease in China. *Progress in Veterinary Medicine,* 30: 89-93.

Nicholson, H. J. (1997). *The Chronicle of the Third Crusade.* Aldershot: Ashgate Publishing.

Nigrovic,L.E. & Wingerter, S.L. (2008, September). Tularemia.*Infect Dis Clin North America*, 22, 3:489-504.

Nuwer, R. (2014, January 1). Ticks Latch On with Telescoping, Barbed Mouthparts.*Scientific American.*

Nuwer, R. (2014, June 5). Lyme Disease's Possible Bacterial Predecessor Found in Ancient Tick. *Scientific American.*

Ogden, N.H., Maarouf, A., Barker, I.K., Bigras-Poulin, M., Lindsay, L.R. (2006). Climate change and the potential for range expansion of the Lyme disease vector *Ixodes scapularis* in Canada. *Int J Parasitol* 36: 63–70.

Olalde, I.,Allentoft, M., Sa´nchez-Quinto, F., Santpere, G., Chiang, C.W.K., DeGiorgio,M., Prado-Martinez, J., Rodrıguez, J.A.Rasmussen, S.,Quilez,J., Ramırez,O.,Marigorta, U.,Fernandez-Callejo, M.,Encina Prada, M., Encinas, J.M.V., Rasmus Nielsen, R., Netea,M., Novembre, J., Sturm,R., Sabeti,P., Marque`s-Bonet,T., Arcadi Navarro,A.,Willerslev, E. & Lalueza-Fox, C. (2014, March 13). Derived immune and ancestral pigmentation alleles in a 7,000-year-old Mesolithic European. *Nature Letter.*

Oorebeek, M. & Kleindorfer, S. (2008). Climate or host availability: what determines the seasonal abundance of ticks. *Parasitol Res,* 103: 871–875.

Oosting, M., Kerstholt, M.,ter Horst,R.,Li, Y.,Deelen, P., Smeekens, S., Jaeger, M., Lachmandas, E.,Vrijmoeth,H., Lupse,M., Flonta, M., Cramer, R.,Kullberg, B., Kumar, V., Xavier,R., Wijmenga,C., Netea, M., Joosten, L.A.B. (2016).Functional and Genomic Architecture of *Borrelia burgdorferi*-Induced Cytokine Responses in Humans. *Cell Host & Microbe.*

Osborne, H.(2015, January 26). New tattoos found on Otzi the Iceman support prehistoric acupuncture theory. *International Business Times.*

Ostfeld, R.& Brunner, J. (2015, February). Climate change and Ixodes tick-borne diseases of humans. *Royal Transactions of the Royal Society B.*

Ostfeld , R., Canham,C.,Oggenfuss, K., Winchcombe, R.& Keesing, (2006, June).Climate, Deer, Rodents, and Acorns as Determinants of Variation in Lyme-Disease Risk. *PLOS,* 4,6:e145.

O'Sullivan, N. J., Teasdale, M. D., Mattiangeli, V., Maixner, F., Pinhasi, R., Bradley, D.G.; Zink,A. (2016, August 18). A whole mitochondria analysis of the Tyrollean Iceman's leather provides insights into the animal sources of Copper Age clothing. *Scientific Reports.*

Ottoni. C., Van Neer ,W., De Cupere, B., Daligault, J., Guimaraes, S., Peters, J., Spassov, N., Prendergast, M.E., Boivin, N., Morales-Muñiz, A., Bălăşescu, A., Becker, C., Benecke, N., Boroneant, A., Buitenhuis, H., Chahoud ,J., Crowther, A., Llorente, L., Manaseryan, N., Monchot, H., Onart, V., Osypińska, M., Putelat, O., Quintana Morales, E.M., Studer, J., Wierer, U., Decorte, R., Grange, T. & Geigl, E. (2017, June 19). The paleogenetics of cat dispersal in the ancient world. *Nature Ecology & Evolution,* 1:0139.

Pan, L., Chen, Z., Huang, Y., Chen, Y., Yu, E. (1996). Investigation on the Host Animal and Transmission Vector of Lyme Disease in Fujian Province. *Chinese Journal of Vector Biology and Control,* 6: 437-439.

Paddock, C.D., Sumner, J.W., Comer, J.A., Zaki, S.R., Goldsmith CS, et al. (2004).*Rickettsia parkeri:* A newly recognized cause of spotted fever rickettsiosis in the United States. *Clinical Infect Dis,* 38: 805–811.

Paddock, C.D., Yabsley, M.J .(2007). Ecological havoc, the rise of white-tailed deer, and the emergence of *Amblyomma americanum*-associated zoonoses in the United States. *Curr Top Microbiology,* 315: 289–324.

Pappas, S. (2014, May 8). Black Death Survivors. The plague preferentially killed the very old and those already in poor health. *LiveScience.*

Parola, P., Paddock, C.D., Raoult, D. (2005). Tick-borne rickettsioses around the world: emerging diseases challenging old concepts. *Clin Microbiol Review,* 18: 719–756.

Patz, J.A., Campbell-Lendrum, D., Holloway, T., Foley, J.A. (2005).Impact of regional climate change on human health. *Nature,* 438: 310–317.

Paulsen, I.T., Nguyen, L., Sliwinski, M.K., Rabus, R., Saier, M.H. (2000). Microbial genome analyses: comparative transport capabilities in eighteen prokaryotes. *J Mol Biology,* 301: 75–100.

Peavey, C.A., Lane, R.S., Damrow, T. (2000, January).Vector competence of Ixodes angustus (Acari: Ixodidae) for Borrelia burgdorferi sensu stricto. *Exp Appl Acarol,* 24, 1:77-84.

Peng,M-S., Palanichamy,M.G.,Yao,Y-G.,Mitra,B., Cheng,Y-T., Zhao,M., Liu,J., Wang, H-W., Pan,H.,Wang, W-Z.,Zhang, A-M., Zhang,W., Wang,D., Zou,Y., Yang,Y.,Chaudhuri,T.K.Kong, Q-P.& Zhang, Y-P.(2011). Inland post-glacial dispersal in East Asia revealed by mitochondrial haplogroup M. *BMC Biology,*9:2.

Persing, D. H.,Telford, S.R. 3rd, Rys, P.N., Dodge, D.E., White, T.J,. Malawista, S..E., Spielman, A. (1990).Detection of *Borrelia burgdorferi* DNA in museum specimens of *Ixodes dammini* ticks. *Science*, 249, 1420–1423.

Persson, C.P. (2016, September 22).The largest genetic study of cats reveals how our furry friends spread out across Europe, Asia, and Africa, and even hitched a ride aboard Viking ships. *ScienceNordic.*

Peters, J., Lebrasseur, O., Deng ,H.,& Larson, G. (2016). Holocene cultural history of Red jungl fowl (Gallus gallus) and its domestic descendant in East Asia. *Quaternary Science Reviews,* 142:102-119.

Phillipe, C.,Poupon, J.,Jeannel, G-F.,Favier, D., Speranta, D., Popescu,S-M., Weil, R., Moulherat, C., Huynh-Charlier, I., Dorion-Peyronnet, C., Lazar, A-M., Herve, C.& Lorin de la Grandmaison,(2013). The embalmed heart of Richard the Lionheart (1199 A.D.): a biological and anthropological analysis. *Scientific Reports,* 3:1296.

Phillips, J. E. (2017). *The Experience of Sickness and Health during Crusader Campaigns to the Eastern Mediterranean, 1095–1274*. PhD thesis, University of Leeds, U.K.

PHYS.org. (2017, January 19). Iceman Otzi's last meal was 'Stone Age bacon' at https://phys.org/news/2017-01-iceman-oetzi-meal-stone-age.html

Piesman ,J., Mather, T.N., Dammin, G.J., Telford, S.R. III, Lastavica, C.C. (1987). Seasonal variation of transmission risk of Lyme disease and human babesiosis. *Am J Epidemiol,* 126: 1187–1189.

Piller, C. (2016, October 12).The 'Swiss Agent': Long-forgotten research unearths new mystery about Lyme disease. *STAT News.*

Pitlik, S. (2017, September 14). First Lyme Disease Patients in US Were Misdiagnosed with Rheumatic Fever. *CONTAGION. Video at* http://www.contagionlive.com/videos/first-lyme-disease-patients-in-us-were-misdiagnosed-with-rheumatic-fever.

Poinar Jr.,G. (2014). Evolutionary History of Terrestrial Pathogens and Endoparasites as Revealed in Fossils and Subfossils. *Advances in Biology*, Article ID 181353.

Poinar, Jr, G. (2015). Spirochete-like cells in a Dominican amber *Ambylomma* tick (Arachnida: Ixodidae). *International Journal of Paleobiology,* 27,5: 565-570.

Poinar, Jr, G & Poinar, R. (2008). *What bugged the Dinosaurs?* Princeton, N.J.: Princeton University Press.

Polito, V.J. (2012). Effects of patch mosaic burning on tick burden of cattle, tick survival, and tick abundance. *M.S. Thesis*. Oklahoma State University, Oklahoma.

Popovic, N., Djuricic,B.,& Valcic, M.(1993) The importance of Lyme Borreliosis in Veterinary Medicine. *Glad Srp Akad Nauka,* 43: 277-285.

Prüfer, K., de Filippo,C.,Grote1,S.,Mafessoni1,F., Korlević, P., Hajdinjak,M., Vernot, B., Skov, L., Hsieh,P., Peyrégne1, S., Reher,D.,Hopfe,C., Nagel,S., Maricic, T., Fu,Q.,Theunert,C. Rogers, R., Skoglund,P., Chintalapati,M.,Dannemann, M., Nelson,B., Key, F., Rudan, P.,Kućan,Z., Ivan Gušić, I.,Golovanova,L., Doronichev, V., Patterson,N.,Reich,D., Eichler, E., Slatkin,M., Schierup, M., Andrés,A., Kelso, J., Meyer, M., & Pääbo, S. (2017, October 5). A high-coverage Neandertal genome from Vindija Cave in Croatia. *Science*.

Radolf, J., Caimano,M., Stevenson,B., Hu, L. (2012). Of ticks, mice and men: understanding the dual-host lifestyle of Lyme disease spirochaetes. *Nature Reviews Microbiology,* 10: 87–99

Rahn, D. (1991). Lyme disease: Clinical manifestations, diagnosis, and treatment. *Arthritis and Rheumatology*, 20, 4:201-218.

Rasmussen, S., Allentoft, M.E. Nielsen,K.,Orlando,L., Sikora, M.,Sjögren, K-G., Pedersen, A.G.,Schubert, M.,Van Dam, A., Kapel,C.M.O.,Nielsen, H.B., Brunak, S., Avetisyan, P., Epimakhov, A., Khalyapin, M.V.,Gnuni,A., Kriiska,A., Lasak,I., Metspalu, M., Vyacheslav Moiseyev, V., Gromov, A., Pokutta,D., Saag,L.,Varul,L., Yepiskoposyan, L.,Sicheritz-Pontén,T.,Foley, R.,Lahr, M.M.,Nielsen,R., Kristiansen, K., & Willerslev, E. (2015, October 22).Early Divergent Strains of Yersinia pestis in Eurasia 5,000 Years Ago. *Cell*, 163, 3: 571–582.

Rattanavong S., Fournier P. E., Chu V., et al.(2014). Bartonella henselae endocarditis in Laos: 'the unsought will go undetected' *PLoS Neglected Tropical Diseases,* 8, 12, article e3385.

Rice, L. (2015, January 19). I've Lost the Ability to Read and Write. *People Magazine*.

Roberts, D., Carlyon, J.,Theisen, M. & Marconi, R. (2000, April).The bdr Gene Families of the Lyme Disease and Relapsing Fever Spirochetes: Potential Influence on Biology, Pathogenesis, and Evolution. *Microbiology Pathology,* 6, 2.

Roebroeks, W. & Villa, P. (2011).On the earliest evidence for habitual use of fire in Europe. *Proceedings of the National Academy of Sciences,* 108,13:5209-5214.

Rogers, J.& Dieppe P. (1994, September). Is tibiofemoral osteoarthritis in the knee joint a new disease? *Ann Rheum Dis.,* 53,9:612-3.

Rollo, F., Ubaldi,M., Ermini,L. & Marota, I. (2002). Ötzi's last meals: DNA analysis of the intestinal content of the Neolithic glacier mummy from the Alps. *PNAS,* 99, 20:12599.

Ross, V. (2011, June 17).Early Farmers were sicker and shorter than their Forager ancestors. *Discover.*

Rothschild, B., Turner, K.& DeLuca, M. (1988, September 16).Symmetrical Erosive Peripheral Polyarthritis in the Late Archaic Period of Alabama. *Science,* 241, 4872:1498-1501.
Roush, J.K., Manley, P.A., Dueland, J. (1989, Oct 1). Rheumatoid arthritis subsequent to Borrelia burgdorferi infection in two dogs. *Vet Med Association,* 195,7:951-3. Case Reports.

Russell, T.M. & Johnson, B.J. (2013, October).Lyme disease spirochaetes possess an aggrecan-binding protease with aggrecanase activity. *Mol Microbiology,* 90, 2: 228-40.

Saetre,K., Godhwani,N., Maria, M., Patel,D., Wang, G., Li, K., Wormser, G. Nolan, S. Babesiosis After Maternal Infection With Borrelia burgdorferi and Babesia microti. (2017, September 16). *Journal of the Pediatric Infectious Diseases Society.*

Sanchez Clemente N., Ugarte-Gil C. A., Solórzano N. (2012). Bartonella bacilliformis: a systematic review of the literature to guide the Research Agenda for Elimination. PLoS Neglected Tropical Diseases, 6,10, article e1819.

Sallares, R.(2002). *Malaria in Rome: History of Malaria in Ancient Italy*. New York: Oxford University Press.

Sankararaman, S., Mallick, S, Dannemann, M. (2014, January 29). The genomic landscape of Neanderthal ancestry in present-day humans. *Nature*.

Sapi ,E., Bastian, S., Mpoy, C., Scott, S., Rattelle, A., Pabbati, N., Poruri, A., Burugu,D., Theophilus, P., Pham, T., Datar, A., Dhaliwal, N., MacDonald, A., Rossi, M., Sinha,S., Luecke, D.F. (2012, October 24).Characterization of Biofilm Formation by Borrelia burgdorferi In Vitro. *Plos One*.

Saraswathy, K.N., Asghar ,M., Samtani, R., Murry, B., Mondal, P.R., Ghosh, P.K.(2012). Spectrum of MTHFR gene SNPs C677T and A1298C: a study among 23 population groups of India. *MolBiol Reports,* 39,4: 502–31.

Sauer, J.R.,Essenberg, C., Bowman, A.S. (2000, July). Salivary glands in ixodid ticks: control and mechanism of secretion. *Journal of Insect Physiology,* 46,7:1069-1078.

Saunder-Hastings, P. & Krewski, D. (2016, December). Reviewing the History of Pandemic Influenza: Understanding Patterns of Emergence and Transmission. *Pathogens,* 5, 4: 66.

Sawa, H.,Kim, H. L. Kuno,K., Suzuki, S., Gotoh,H.,Takada, M., Takahata,N., Satta, Y. & Akishinonomiya, F. (2010, May 19). Origin and Genetic Variation of Domestic Chickens with Special Reference to Junglefowls *Gallus g. gallus* and *G. various*. *PLOS One,* 5, 5.

Schaller, J. MD & Mountjoy,K. (2012). *What You May Not Know About Bartonella, Babesia, Lyme Disease, and Other Tick & Flea-Borne Infections.* International University Infectious Disease Press.

Schaller, J.(2008). *The Diagnosis, Treatment and Prevention of Bartonella.* Florida: Hope Academy Press.

Schlott ,T., Eiffert, H., Schmidt-Schultz, T., Gebhardt, M., Parzinger, H., Schultz, M.(2007, November-December). Detection and analysis of cancer genes amplified from bone material of a Scythian royal burial in Arzhan near Tuva, Siberia. *Anticancer Research* 27, 6B:4117-9.

Schulze, T.L., Jordan, R.A., Hung ,R.W. (2001). Potential effects of animal activity on the spatial distribution of *Ixodes scapularis* and *Amblyomma americanum* (Acari: Ixodidae). *Environ Entomol* 30: 568–577.

Schuster, F. L. (2002, July).Cultivation of Babesia and Babesia-Like Blood Parasites: Agents of an Emerging Zoonotic Disease. *Clinical Microbiology Re*view 15, 3: 365–373.

Schwartzman,W.A., Patnaik, M.,Singer,E. & Visscher,B.(1998). Features of Bartonella-associated HIV dementias. *Abstracts of the 5th Conference on Retroviruses and Opportunistic Infections*, Chicago, IL.

Seifert, S., Khatchikian, C., Zhou,W., & Brisson, D. (April 2015).Evolution and population genomics of the Lyme borreliosis pathogen, Borrelia burgdorferi. *Ticks and Tick-borne diseases,* 6:344-351.

Seth A., Raina U., Thirumalai S., Batta S., Ghosh B.(2015). Full-thickness macular hole in Bartonella henselae neuroretinitis in an 11-year-old girl. *Oman Journal of Ophthalmology*, 8,1:44–46.
SIGMA Type 2 Diabetes Consortium. (2013). Sequence variants in SLC16A11 are a common risk factor for type 2 diabetes in Mexico. *Nature.*

Silver, H. (1997, March 1). Lyme Disease during Pregnancy. *Infectious Disease Clinics of North America,*11, 1: 93-97.

Solecki, R. S. (1954). Shanidar cave: a paleolithic site in northern Iraq. *Annual Report of the Smithsonian Institution:*389–425.

Solecki, R.S.(1975).Shanidar IV, a Neanderthal Flower Burial in Northern Iraq. *Science*, 190, 4217: 880-881.

Solecki, R. S. & Agelarakis, A. (2004). *The Proto-Neolithic Cemetery in Shanidar Cave*. Texas A&M University Press.

Soucheray, S. (2013, December 5). Bartonella is everywhere. What don't we know more about it? *North Carolina Health News*.

Sparks, J.C., Masters,R.E., Engle, D.M., Palmer, M.W., Michael ,W. (1998). Effects of late growing-season and late dormant-season prescribed fire on herbaceous vegetation in restored pine-grassland communities. *J Veg Sci,* 9: 133–142.

Stafford III, K.C., Ward, J.S., Magnarelli, L.A. (1998). Impact of controlled burns on the abundance of *Ixodes scapularis* (Acari: Ixodidae). *J Med Entomology,* 35: 510–513.

Steele, V. (2005). *Bleed, Blister and Purge: A History of Medicine on the American Frontier.* Missoula, Montana: Mountain Press Publishing Company.

Storey, A.A., Quiroz, D., Beavan, N., and Matisoo-Smith, E. (2013). Polynesian chickens in the New World: a detailed application of a commensal approach. *Archaeology in Oceania* 48,2:101-119.

Stricker, R.B. and Fesler, M.C. (2017, May 3). Chronic Lyme Disease: A Working Case Definition. *Chronic Diseases International* 4,1: 1025.

Strickland, A. (1868). *Lives of the Queens of England, from the Norman Conquest, 2*. Bell Publishing.

Stromdahl, E.Y. & Hickling, G.J. (2012). Beyond Lyme: etiology of tick-borne human diseases with emphasis on the South-Eastern United States. *Zoonoses Public Health,* 59: 48–64.

Sun, Y., Rongman, X.& Cao, W. (2003). Ixodes sinensis: Competence as a vector to transmit the Lyme disease spirochete Borrelia garinii. *Vector Borne Zoonotic Disease,* 1: 39-44.

Szécsényi-Nagy, A., Brandt, G., Keer, V. , Jakucs, J., Haak, W. ,Möller-Rieker, S. , Kitti Köhler, K. , Gusztáv Mende, B., Fecher, M., Oross, K. , Marton,T. , Osztás, A., Kiss, V. , Pál, G.fi , Molnár,E. , K Sebők, K., Czene,A., Paluch,T. , Šlaus, M. , Novak, M. , Pećina- Šlaus, N. , Ősz, B., Voicsek, V., Somogyi, K. , Tóth,G., Kromer, B., Bánffy, E., Alt,K.W. (2015, April 22). Tracing the genetic origin of Europe's first farmers reveals insights into their social organization. *Proceedings B of The Royal Society,* 282,1805.

Tang, T.T., Zhang, L., Bansal, A., Grynpas, M.& Moriarty, T.J. (2016,December 12).The Lyme disease pathogen Borrelia burgdorferi infects murine bone and induces trabecular bone loss. *Infect Immun.*

Taviner, M., Thwaites, G., Gant, V. (1998). The English Sweating Sickness, 1485-1551:A Viral Pulmonary Disease? *Medical History,* 42:96-98.

Than, K. (2011, June 23). Iceman's stomach full of goat meat. *National Geographic.*

Thio, C., Astemborski, J., Bashiroval, A., Mosbruger, T., Greer, S., Witt, M., Goedert, J., Hilgartner, M., Majeske, A., O'Brien, S., Thomas, D., & Carrington, M. (2007). Genetic Protection against Hepatitis B Virus Conferred by CCR5Δ32. *Journal Virology,* 81, 2: 441-445.

Thomas, L., Jr. (2013, July 25). Burning Questions: Can Fire Reduce Tick Abundance? *Quality Deer Management.*

Thomas, R.J., Dumler, J.S. & Carolyn, J.A. (2009). Current management of human granulocytic anaplasmosis, human monocytic ehrlichiosis, and *Ehrlichia ewingii* ehrlichiosis. *Expert Rev Anti Infect Ther,* 7: 709–722.

Thomson,V., Lebrasseur, O., Austin, J.J., Hunt, T.L., Burney, D.A., Denham, T., Rawlence, N.J., Wood, J.R., Gongora, J., Girdland Flink, L.(2014). Using ancient DNA to study the origins and dispersal of ancestral Polynesian chickens across the Pacific. *PANS* 111,13: 4826-4831.

Tierney, J. & Zander, P. (2017). A climatic context for the out-of-Africa migration: Humans migrated out of Africa as the climate shifted from wet to very dry about 6000 years ago. *Geology.*

Townes, G. & Owensby, C. (1984). Long-term effects of annual burns at different dates in ungrazed Kansas tallgrass prairie. *J Range Manage,* 37: 392–397.

Tripp, S. (2014). *Prescribed Fire and Deer Ticks: A Management Method for the Primary Vector of Lyme Disease in the Eastern United States.* Master of the Arts Thesis. Binghamton University, SUNY.

Turbervile, G.(1576). *The Book of Hunting.*

Twomey, T. (February 2013). The Cognitive Implications of Controlled Fire Use by Early Humans, *Cambridge Archeological Journal,* 23, 1:113-128.

Uilenberg, G.(2006, May 31). Babesia--a historical overview.*Vet Parasitology,*138,1-2:3-10.
Unknown. (2008, September 25). Bill Chinnock Obituary. *Bangor Daily News.*

Valtuena, A.A., Mittnik,A., Massy,K.,Allmae, R., Daubaras, M., Jankauskas,R.,Torv,M., Pfrengle,S., Spyrou,M., Feldman,M., Haak, W., Bos, K., Stockhammer, P., Alexander, Herbig, A.&

Krause, J.(2016, December).The Stone Age Plague: 1000 years of plague in Eurasia. *Cold Spring Harbor Preprint.*

van Hoofa, T., Frans, P., Bunnik, M., Jean G.M.,Wolfram, W., Kürschnera, M.Visschera, H. (2006, August 4). Forest re-growth on medieval farmland after the Black Death pandemic.Implications for atmospheric CO2 levels. *Palaeogeography, Palaeoclimatology, Palaeoecology*, 237, 2–4:396-409.

Vannier, E.,Gerwurz, B.E.,Krause,P.J. (2008, September). Human babesiosis. *Infectious Dis Clin North America* 22, 3:469-88.

Varlik, N. (2017). *Plague and Contagion in the Islamic Mediterranean.* High Wycombe,U.K.:ARC Humanities Press.

Vigne, J., Evin,A., Cucchi,T., Dai,L., Yu, C.,Hu,S.,Soulages,N., Wang,W.,Sun,Z.,Gao,J.,Dobney,K., Yuan, J. (2016, January). Earliest "Domestic" Cats in China Identified as Leopard Cat (*Prionailurus bengalensis*). *PLOS ONE.*

Waldron, T. (1995). Changes in the distribution of osteoarthritis over historical time.*International Journal Osteoarchaeoly,*5:385–9. Wallace,I.,Worthington,S.,Felson,D.T.,Jurmaind,R.,Wrene, K., Maijanenf,H.,Woods,R.& Liebermana, D.(2017, August 29). Knee osteoarthritis has doubled in prevalence since the mid-20th century. *PNAS,* 114, 35: 9332–9336.

Walter, K.S., Carpi, G., Caccone,A., Diuk-Wasser, M.(2017, August). Insights into the ancient spread of Lyme disease across North America. *Nature Ecology and Evolution 1:* 1569-1576.

Wang, S., Xu, X., Shrestha, N., Zimmermann, N., Tang, Z.,Wang, Z. (2017). Response of spatial vegetation distribution in China to climate changes since the Last Glacial Maximum (LGM). *Plos One.*

Wang, Y.Y., Li, J., Wang, S., Hu, M.& Lu, F.L. (2011). Tick-borne infectious diseases. *Infectious Disease Information,* 1: 58-61.

Weber, K, Bratzke, HJ, Neubert, U, Wilske, B,& Duray, PH.(1988, April 7). Borrelia burgdorferi in a newborn despite oral penicillin for Lyme borreliosis during pregnancy. *Pediatr Infect Dis J.* 7,4 : 286-9.

Wells, S. (2004). *The Journey of Man: A Genetic Odyssey.* New York: Random House.

Wheelis, M. (2002, September).Warfare at the 1346 Siege of Caffa. Origin of the 14th-Century Pandemic Historical Background to the Siege of Caffa Gabriele de' Mussi The Narrative of Gabriele De' Mussi. *Emerging Infectious Disease*, 8: 9.

White, N. J. (July 1997). Assessment of the pharmacodynamic properties of antimalarial drugs in vivo. *Antimicrob. Agents Chemother,* 41, 7: 1413–22.

Whitmire,W.M.. & Garon, C.F.(1993, April). Specific and nonspecific responses of murine B cells to membrane blebs of Borrelia burgdorferi. *Infect Immunity* I61,4:1460-7.

Williams, M. (2000). Dark ages and dark areas: global deforestation in the deep past. *Journal of Historical Geography,* 26, 1: 28–46.

Williams, M. (2008). A New Look at Global Forest Histories of Land Clearing. *The Annual Review of Environment and Resources.*

Willis, A.A., Widmann, R.F., Flynn, J.M., Green, D.W.& Onel, K.B.(2003). Lyme arthritis presenting as acute septic arthritis in children. *J Pediatr Orthopedics* 23,1:114–118.

Willis, D., Carter, R., Murdock, C., & Blair, B. (2012). Relationship between habitat type, fire frequency, and *Amblyomma americanum*, populations in east-central Alabama. *Journal Vector Ecology* 37: 373–381.

Wilson, M. (1986). Reduced abundance of adult *Ixodes dammini* (Acari: Ixodidae) following destruction of vegetation. *Journal of Economic Entomology* 79: 693–696.

Wu, G.H.& Jiang, Z.K. (2007). Lyme disease and prevention and control of ticks. *Chinese Journal of Hygienic Insecticides*, 5: 312-314.

Wu, X-B., Na,R-H., Wei,S-S., Zhu, J-S.& Peng, H-J. (2013, April 23). Distribution of tick-borne diseases in China. *Parasites & Vectors*.

Xiang, H, Gao, J, Yu, B, Zhou, H, Cai, D, Zhang, Y, Chen, X, Wang, X, Hofreiter, M, and Zhao, X. (2014). Early Holocene chicken domestication in northern China. *Proceedings of the National Academy of Sciences* 111,49:17564-17569.

Yakub, M., Moti, N., Parveen, S., Chaudhry, B.& AzamI,I. (2012).Polymorphisms in MTHFR, MS and CBS genes and homocysteine levels in a Pakistani population.*PLOS ONE*, 7,3.

Yan, S., Wang, C-C., Zheng, H-X., Wang, W., Qin, Z-D., Wei, L-H., (2014, August 29).Y Chromosomes of 40% Chinese Descend from Three Neolithic Super-Grandfathers. *PLOS ONE*, 9,8.

Yang, M., Gao,X.,Theunert, C., Tong, H., Aximu-Petri, A., Nickel,B.,Slatkin, M., Meyer, M., Pääbo, S., J Kelso, J., Fu, Q. (In Press 2017) 40,000-Year-Old Individual from Asia Provides Insight into Early Population Structure in Eurasia. *Current Biology*.

Young, S. (2017, May 22). Alec Baldwin Opens Up About Suffering From Lyme Disease and Thinking He Was Going to Die. *People Magazine*.

Zhang, D. (2007). *The Legend of Mawangdui*. Hunan Sheng, China: Changsa.

Zhang, J-M, et al. (2007).Cytokines, Inflammation and Pain. *International Anesthesiology Clinics*, 45, 2:27-37.

Zhang, QC.& Zhang, Y.(2006). *Lyme Disease and Modern Chinese Medicine.* Sino-Med Research Institute.

Zhang, S.(2017, April 6). The Scientist Who Stumbled Upon a Tick Full of 20-Million-Year-Old Blood. He's the same scientist who inspired Jurassic Park. *The Atlantic.*

Zlobin, V., Pogodina, V., Kahl, O.(2017, October). A brief history of the discovery of tick-borne encephalitis virus in the late 1930s (based on reminiscences of members of the expeditions, their colleagues, and relatives) *Ticks and Tick-borne Diseases*, 8, 6: 813-820.

Also by M.M. Drymon

Disguised as the Devil: How Lyme Disease Created Witches and Changed History.

Scotch-Irish Folkways in America.

A Place Called Crockett's Corner.

Cover Illustrations:
Front- *Spirochetes* by Scivit.
Back- Catherine of Aragon by M. Sittow, circa 1500-1505. Ancient *Ixodes* tick in amber, courtesy, Dr. George Poinar, Jr., Oregon State University.

www.ingramcontent.com/pod-product-compliance
Lightning Source LLC
Chambersburg PA
CBHW021356210526
45463CB00001B/122